REVERSING
HEALTH RISKS

REVERSING HEALTH RISKS

HOW TO GET OUT OF THE HIGH-RISK CATEGORY FOR CANCER, HEART DISEASE, DIABETES, AND OTHER HEALTH PROBLEMS

Julian Whitaker, M.D.

&

June Roth, M.S.

G. P. Putnam's Sons/New York

G. P. Putnam's Sons
Publishers Since 1838
200 Madison Avenue
New York, NY 10016

Library of Congress Cataloging-in-Publication Data

Whitaker, Julian M.
Reversing health risks / by Julian Whitaker & June Roth.—1st
American ed.

p. cm.
Includes index.
1. Chronic diseases—Prevention.   2. Blood—Analysis.   3. Health
status indicators.   4. Nutrition.   5. Health.   I. Roth, June, date.
II. Title.
RC108.W45   1988
616.07'561—dc19   88-12212 CIP
ISBN 0-399-13396-8

Printed in the United States of America
1   2   3   4   5   6   7   8   9   10

*This book is dedicated to all those who
would like to understand what their blood
tests actually reveal, who would like to
participate in preventing potential
degenerative disease, who would like to
communicate better with their doctors,
and who would like to take an active role
in improving their wellness profile.*

Contents

CONTENTS

Introduction

No other component of the body receives as much attention as the blood. If you are sick, one of the first things the physician will do is run a battery of blood tests, looking for clues to the diagnosis. Oftentimes these blood tests alone provide the answer. Moreover, routine physical examinations almost always include a series of blood tests, and during a hospital stay, various blood tests may be done daily.

Most major health concerns—heart disease, AIDS, high blood pressure, diabetes—are directly related to constituents that can be measured in the blood. Such terms as blood-cholesterol level, blood-sugar level, and white blood count pop up in conversation regularly, yet most people, even those who are knowledgeable about health, know very little about the various blood tests that are markers for disease, much less about how to improve the results of the tests in order to avoid those diseases.

This book addresses that very subject and offers a program designed to achieve and maintain blood tests in the normal range. Health is not simply the absence of disease, but indicates that all systems of the body are working smoothly, efficiently, and harmoniously.

There are millions of men and women in this country in ill health without a specifically diagnosed disease. In Western medicine, physicians generally ignore individuals in poor health, offering them no services unless a well-recognized disease pattern occurs. The most glaring example of this would be heart disease. Often physicians will spend many years neglecting patients with elevated cholesterol levels, which we shall see is a direct indicator of impending heart disease. When the heart attack finally occurs, the physician springs into action with expensive technology. Prevention should start when the first blood warnings appear.

This book outlines a program to obtain and maintain maximum health by calling early attention to abnormal blood-test results. There are three aspects to correcting blood warnings before they have a chance to develop into a full-blown disease: diet, exercise, and vitamins and minerals.

Your first line of defense is an appropriate diet, which is responsible for more changes in the blood chemistry than any other factor. Excessive fat and cholesterol in the diet markedly elevate the blood-cholesterol and blood-fat levels, increasing the chance of a heart attack. Inadequate amounts of carbohydrates and fiber in the diet decrease the body's sensitivity to insulin, and the blood-sugar level begins to elevate in the blood, heralding a diabetic condition. Excessive protein often causes an elevation in the blood level of uric acid, which indicates an increased risk not only for gouty arthritis, but also for heart disease and kidney stones. The rich American diet, high in fat and animal protein, may cause slight elevations in the white blood count, which have recently been found to be another measurable risk factor for heart disease.

These dangerous changes in the blood chemistry can be avoided and reversed with basic changes in the diet, primarily in the composition of the calories consumed. Recent research indicates that most of the calories should come from vegetable foods that are high in complex carbohydrates. When a dietary pattern emphasizes fat or protein calories, the various energy-producing systems in the body begin to break down, the blood chemistry is altered, and disease is on the way.

Your second line of defense is exercise. The old adage of "use it or lose it" is certainly more true than we would care to believe. Almost all biological systems, with the exception of modern man, and certainly most mammals, live as a result of physical exertion. For instance, predators, such as lions and tigers, must stalk and run down their prey, and more vegetarian mammals are constantly on the move in search of food. Only modern man lives as a result of intellectual activity and no longer has to expend physical energy to find food for survival. However, easy access to food has caused a sedentary lifestyle. Cultural advancement has become a major reason for the ill health that is so prevalent in our modern society.

There are two forms of exercise. The first and most important is aerobic conditioning. Aerobic conditioning means moving the body through space, exercising the large muscle groups and the cardiovascular system. This form of exercise consumes copious amounts of energy. The second form of exercise is strength conditioning—working out with weights or resistance machines that strengthen and tone the muscle groups of the body.

Regular exercise alters the blood chemistry in numerous beneficial ways. For example, it enhances the way the body clears fat from the blood, so as a result the triglyceride level almost always drops. Exercise also increases the level of HDL (see chapter 2), which significantly reduces the risk of heart attack. Furthermore, exercise tends to maintain the blood in a more fluid state, thus reducing the risk of abnormal blood-clot formation. When tiny blood clots do form, those who exercise regularly are able to clear the blood of these clots more rapidly.

Your third line of defense against degenerative disease is the utilization of vitamins and minerals. Essential to optimal nutrition is the optimal intake of micronutrients, including vitamins, minerals, and trace elements. These substances are the keys to optimal function of all energy-producing systems in our bodies.

This book explores research that goes beyond the concept of eliminating vitamin and mineral deficiency, showing how to supplement your diet with the optimal amount of micronutrients for optimal health.

An obvious criticism of nutritional supplements is that a natural diet should provide all of the vitamins, minerals, and trace elements for good health, and that supplementation is not necessary. However, that position gives little regard to how personal lifestyle and habits interact with the nutrients in your food. In fact, if you eat on the run, are under stress, smoke, drink alcoholic beverages, and use one or more medications, it is highly likely that your nutrient bank is in a constant state of depletion. In addition, as Dr. Roger Williams, the discoverer of pantothenic acid, pointed out over thirty years ago, we all are biologically different with wide variations in our needs for specific nutrients. Supplementation acts to insure the optimal amounts of nutrients for optimal health.

Alterations in blood-chemistry levels are less predictable with nutritional supplements than they are with diet and exercise changes, primarily because we are all different, as are the changes brought on by the intake of nutrients.

For instance, increased intake of vitamin C has been shown to lower the blood cholesterol in some but not in others. This is also true for supplementation with chromium. Some studies show that vitamin E will elevate the HDL level of the blood, while others show that it has no effect. Niacin, however, in large doses, is a reliable and safe method of lowering the blood levels of cholesterol and triglycerides, and elevating the HDL cholesterol level.

The rationale for taking supplements is to prevent the possibility of inadequate intake of these nutrients, thus insuring optimal function of the metabolic systems of the body.

This book shows you how to maintain a normal blood profile, avoid nutritional bankruptcy, and keep your body in fit condition to be able to thrive and stay alive. You are going to learn how to understand all of the blood tests that can predict problems long before they occur. This book gives you all the tools that are currently known to improve blood chemistry, so you can become a true partner in your physical well-being.

Does this program work?

Well, for Rolly Pulaski it worked, and continues to.

In September of 1986, this very pleasant and successful fifty-one-year-old architect came to the Whitaker Wellness Institute hoping for a different approach to his long-standing problem with high blood pressure. Over the last thirty years he had taken almost every medication available for lowering blood pressure. However, his blood pressure remained in the high-normal range even on medication, and when first seen he was taking Hydrochlorothiazide, 50 milligrams per day, and Lopressor, a particularly powerful medication, 100 milligrams twice a day. He weighed 223 pounds, and wanted to slim down.

We told Mr. Pulaski at that time we had no cures for his problem but would put him on a program that, we hoped, would not only reduce his reliance on high-blood-pressure medication, but also improve his general health and reduce the risk for other problems as well. In addition, we told him that we would follow his progress by using a complete blood panel on a regular basis and would alter our approach with him based upon those changes.

Initially, on medication, his blood pressure was 195/90. On September 23, 1986 his blood profile was as follows:

Total cholesterol	263
HDL cholesterol	36
Cholesterol:HDL ratio	7.3
Fasting glucose	96
Uric acid	6.7
Triglyceride	175

He was put on the type of diet outlined in part II of this book and began an exercise regimen consisting primarily of walking.

On January 9, 1987, he weighed 199½ pounds, his blood-cholesterol level had dropped to 204, his HDL had increased to 43, his cholesterol:HDL ratio had increased to 4.7, his fasting glucose was down to 88, uric acid to 6.0, and his triglyceride had dropped all the way to 79. His blood pressure at that time was 130/82. When we submitted his initial data to the computer, his cardiac risk was quite high, but by January 9, three and a half months later, his cardiac risk had dropped substantially.

The changes he is now experiencing in his lifestyle measurably reduce his risk of other diseases as well. In addition, his sense of well-being has increased, and he has become a "zealot" for health.

We wish you similar success!

JUNE ROTH, M.S.
Teaneck, New Jersey

JULIAN M. WHITAKER, M.D.
Whitaker Wellness Institute
Newport Beach, California

PART I

YOUR BLOOD CHEMISTRY AND WHAT IT REVEALS

—— 1 ——

Blood and Its Components

Blood may not be the essence of life, but the common use of the word in language is testimony to the importance of blood: "That account is the life-blood of this business"; "It was a bloody revolution"; "Blood was spilled"; "Hot blood"; "Cold blood."

Tests on blood provide us with the portal through which we can see health or disease coming or going and upon which we can base an action program to prevent disease. Knowledge of your body's blood chemistry is your best defense against degenerative disease. Blood tests can indicate what is happening long before any symptoms of disease occur. Indeed, your blood profile is one of the best screening devices now known to medicine. When blood tests reveal slight abnormalities, it is urgent to reverse the warnings as quickly as possible to avert the danger of degenerative disease. When you understand these tests and the role blood plays in your body, you can keep your test scores within normal ranges through diet, exercise, and proper vitamin and mineral intake. We tend to take blood for granted, yet the quality of your blood will ultimately affect the quality of your life.

Blood is made up of both cellular and liquid components. The cellular component of blood contains red blood cells, white blood cells, and platelets. Blood is the rapid transit system of the body, efficiently transporting all manner of products. After the food we eat is broken down into its component parts, it is carried by the blood to the liver and other parts of the body. Hormones manufactured in various glands are carried by the blood to the organs that are affected by them. The blood functions as the carrier for both negative and positive elements. Every component of our bodies has at one time been transported or utilized by the blood.

RED BLOOD CELLS

Red blood cells are carriers of oxygen. They measure approximately 1/10,000th of an inch in diameter and give blood its red color. These cells, which contain hemoglobin, pick up oxygen in the lungs, transport it to the cells, and carry back carbon dioxide to be expelled by the lungs.

Red blood cells make up approximately 40 percent of the volume of blood and are continually produced in the bone marrow. All the bones of our skeleton contain a dense, hard outer layer that serves as the structural support of our bodies, as well as a soft, spongy inner core—the bone marrow. The number of red blood cells produced is determined in reverse proportion to the quantity of oxygen that is transported by the blood to the cells of the body. If there is significant blood loss, reducing the number of red blood cells and in turn reducing the amount of oxygen that is transported throughout the body, the body will react by rapidly increasing the production of red blood cells. In addition, if someone from sea level travels to higher altitudes, where the available oxygen in the air is less, there will be an increased production of red blood cells as well.

The principal factor that stimulates this red-blood-cell production is a hormone called erythropoietin. Ninety to ninety-five percent of this hormone is produced by the kidney, which contains sensors that constantly monitor the available oxygen in the blood. When the oxygen level falls, erythropoietin is produced, immediately stimulating the bone marrow to increase production of red blood cells. When the transport of oxygen is adequate, erythropoietin production falls and red-blood-cell production follows suit.

This system of control of red-blood-cell production by the bone marrow is very powerful. If the kidney is producing substantial amounts of erythropoietin in response to reduced oxygen-carrying capacity of the blood, the bone marrow is capable of producing red blood cells at ten times its normal rate. On the other hand, if more than adequate oxygen is being supplied by the blood, the production of erythropoietin can drop to almost zero and the bone marrow can literally shut down its production of red blood cells to a similar level.

The normal red blood cell has a life span of about 120 days. As the red blood cell ages, its covering membrane becomes more fragile and the cell becomes less pliable. In its normal course through the body, the red blood cell goes through small capillaries, often smaller in diameter than the cell itself, so that older red blood cells rupture. This is particularly true in the spleen, which, with its particularly small capillaries, acts as the graveyard for most old red blood cells. In the spleen, the component parts of the ruptured cells are immediately saved for the production of new cells. The destruction of old red blood cells occurs throughout the body as well, but when the spleen is removed, the number of old red blood cells circulating in the body goes up considerably.

Anemia

Anemia represents a deficiency of red blood cells that occurs either by too rapid a loss of red blood cells or inadequate production.

Overly rapid loss of red blood cells occurs with acute or chronic bleeding. The blood loss exceeds the body's ability to replace red blood cells. Often this form of blood-loss anemia indicates another disease. For instance, there can be both acute and chronic losses of blood in the gastrointestinal tract. Men and women who suffer with ulcers or cancer of the stomach or of the intestinal tract will often lose substantial amounts of blood that can go undetected for weeks or months. The body may not be able to keep up with this rate of blood loss, and the amount of red blood cells circulating in the blood decreases.

Occasionally, women who have excessive menstrual flow will develop anemia if they lose more iron in the blood than is taken in the diet. This is not common but does occur.

The red-blood-cell count will drop if the production of red blood cells in the bone marrow decreases. This is called *aplastic anemia*. For instance, individuals exposed to intense radiation, either from a nuclear accident or as a form of therapy for cancer, have marked reduction in bone-marrow activity, which can be fatal in a few weeks.

Another form of anemia occurs from absence of vitamin B_{12} or of folic acid. The anemia of B_{12} deficiency, called *pernicious* or *megaloblastic anemia*, is not caused by B_{12} deficiency in the diet, but rather the inability to absorb vitamin B_{12} through the stomach. The stomach produces gastric acid necessary for B_{12} production, as well as an "intrinsic factor" necessary for vitamin B_{12} absorption. If gastric-acid production is reduced in the stomach, then the intrinsic factor is reduced. Without B_{12}, the natural process of cell division and red-blood-cell production falls.

Another form of reduced red-blood-cell concentration in the blood is increase in red-blood-cell destruction. This is called *hemolytic anemia*. Many forms of hemolytic anemia are inherited, the most common being *sickle-cell anemia*, found in .3 to 1 percent of American blacks. This form of anemia is caused by an abnormal protein in the hemoglobin that increases the fragility of the red blood cell and rapidly increases red-blood-cell destruction. When red blood cells containing the abnormal sickle-cell-anemia protein are exposed to slightly reduced oxygen concentrations, the red blood cell "sickles," dramatically changing its shape from a circular cell that looks like a dinner plate to a fragile, elongated, sicklelike structure. As their flow characteristics are altered, these cells are rapidly destroyed in the body.

WHITE BLOOD CELLS

White blood cells make up an additional cellular component of the blood, but their number is extremely small compared to the red blood cells contained in blood. While the red blood cells account for approximately 40 percent of the volume of whole blood, the white blood cells account for far less than one percent. Whereas the number of red blood cells normally ranges around 4.7 to 5.2 *million* per cubic millimeter, there are generally only five to ten *thousand* white blood cells per cubic millimeter. White blood cells, as a group called leukocytes, are the mobile units of the body's immune system. Their concentration increases with almost any form of disease, particularly infectious diseases. They rapidly accumulate in areas of the body that are infected and do battle with the offending agent, whether it is a virus or bacteria.

There are five types of white blood cells in the following percentages:

Polymorphonuclear Neutrophils	60–65%
Polymorphonuclear Eosinophils	2–4%
Polymorphonuclear Basophils	.5–1.5%
Lymphocytes	25–35%
Monocytes	5.3%

Polymorphonuclear Neutrophils

Neutrophils, by far the most commonly found white blood cell, are the front-line foot soldiers of the defense system. They are rapidly attracted to and then phagocytize (engulf) any bacteria or foreign body material contained in the blood. These white blood cells contain strong enzymes in small packets inside the cell that destroy the foreign or offending particle. Neutrophils continue to phagocytize the foreign matter until the enzyme destroys all of the engulfed particles and the white blood cell itself. If there is substantial infection or debris, this process of engulfing and destroying particles and cells produces a viscous material, commonly known as pus.

When there is active infection in the body, the number of white blood cells as well as the percentage of polymorphonuclear neutrophils significantly increases. For instance, someone suffering from appendicitis will characteristically have a white blood cell count of 15–20,000, with 90 to 95 percent of the white blood cells polymorphonuclear neutrophils or "band cells." Band cells are simply very young polymorphonuclear neutrophils that have been released by the bone marrow even before maturation to do battle with the offending agent.

Polymorphonuclear Eosinophils

Eosinophils are weak phagocytes, meaning they do not generally engulf smaller particles. However, they are produced in large quantities and their percentage in the blood increases dramatically in men and women who suffer with parasite infections. Parasites include amoeba cells that infest various tissues of the body, as well as worms that live in the gastrointestinal tract. These offending agents are too large to be phagocytized by the much smaller white blood cells. The eosinophil, however, can attach itself to the parasite and release substances that can kill many of them.

In addition, in patients that suffer from allergic reaction, there is an increase in eosinophil percentage in the blood. This is because in areas where there is allergic response, such as in the lungs of patients who have asthma, there is an increased concentration of eosinophils that detoxify some of the products of inflammation brought on by the allergic attack.

Basophils

Basophils occur in small percentages in the blood but play an increasingly important role in allergic reactions. When the body responds to an offending agent that stimulates an allergic reaction, the basophil will release histamine, bradykinin, serotonin, and heparin. The substances will cause local constriction of the blood cell and the wheezing associated with an asthma attack.

21

Lymphocytes

Lymphocytes are another type of the body's soldiers of immunity. If the polymorphonuclear neutrophils are the foot soldiers in the body's defense system, the lymphocytes would be the pilots, or navy captains, that fight disease by dropping bombs, or shooting large guns across distances. The lymphocytes produce antibodies that circulate in the blood and attack the offending agent (antigen).

There are two distinct forms of lymphocytes, T lymphocytes and B lymphocytes. T lymphocytes derive their name from the thymus gland, where they are first processed, generally before birth. Their function is that of cellular immunity (the growth of special white blood cells after exposure to a foreign substance). T cells "remember" previous exposure to specific antigens, and can produce antibodies for future encounters. The cell travels to the antigen, where the antibody is released.

The additional lymphocytes are known as B lymphocytes, and their function is that of humoral immunity (the development and continuing presence of circulating antibodies). In response to a specific antigen, these lymphocytes release a specific antibody into the blood.

In patients with AIDS, there is significant alteration in the function of lymphocytes, as well as all the other aspects of the body's immune system.

Monocytes

Monocytes look like very large lymphocytes. Like neutrophils, these cells undergo phagocytic activity. However, a monocyte circulating in the blood is an immature cell that must migrate out of the bloodstream into the tissues, where it swells to ten times its previous size. This very large cell is now called a macrophage, and is capable of phagocytizing much larger particles.

PLATELETS

In addition to the various types of red and white cells, the third cellular component of the blood is platelets. Platelets are very small, sandlike particles, approximately one-third the size of a red blood cell. They number 150 to 350 thousand per cubic millimeter of blood, functioning primarily in the formation of blood clots to control or stop blood loss.

If a small blood vessel is punctured, platelets will immediately adhere to the area of damage in the blood vessel. If the rupture of the blood vessel is very small, all that is needed to control blood loss is a platelet plug. If the rupture in the blood vessel is very large, then platelets combine with red blood cells to form a blood clot. For blood clotting to occur, there is a cascade of reactions that involve twelve specific factors, including platelets. A hemophiliac, or a bleeder, has a genetically derived deficiency of factor 8 in the bloodclotting cascade. These individuals require periodic replacement of factor 8 or are susceptible to uncontrollable bleeding. For them, a sprained ankle or a small cut is a medical emergency.

Platelets are formed in the bone marrow from megakaryocytes (very large cells which do not themselves leave the bone marrow). Small platelets are formed on the surface of these large cells, are pinched off, then released into the blood. If platelet production is decreased and the platelet count in the blood drops below 100 thousand per cubic millimeter, the condition is called thrombocytopenia. If the platelet count is between 40 thousand and 100 thousand per cubic millimeter, spontaneous bleeding does not occur, but excessive bleeding may occur with injury or surgery. With a platelet count below 40 thousand per cubic millimeter, spontaneous bleeding is common. This form of bleeding results in small petechiae (best described as "pinpoint bruises"), larger bruises called purpuric spots, and rather severe bruises called confluent ecchymoses. With a very low platelet count, bleeding is very common from the gums in the mouth, or from the cellular surfaces of the nose, uterus, gastrointestinal tract, urinary tract, or respiratory tracts in the lung.

Thrombocytopenia, or low platelets, can occur from a variety of causes. In most cases thrombocytopenia is idiopathic, meaning no known cause can be determined. Generally, 80 percent of those who have this disorder will recover regardless of therapy. If the condition persists, various forms of treatment are available, including the administration of steroid hormones, removal of the spleen (which reduces destruction of platelets in the bloodstream), and transfusion of platelets.

TESTING THE CELLULAR COMPONENTS OF BLOOD

The cellular components of the blood are tested from a sample of the blood that contains an anticlotting factor. This factor prevents the cellular components from becoming involved in a blood clot that would prevent their examination.

The *hematocrit*, or percentage of the volume of blood taken up by the red blood cells, is measured by contrifuging (rapidly spinning) a tube of unclotted blood. All of the red blood cells and other cellular components of the blood migrate to the bottom of the tube, leaving the plasma (a clear, yellowish liquid) at the top. Normally, the pack of red blood cells and other cellular components account for 38 to 45 percent of the total volume of blood after centrifugation. If there is anemia, or significant reduction in the red-blood-cell component of the blood, the hematocrit will drop to the low thirties, twenties, or even into the teens. Other evaluations of the cellular components of blood are made by observing a small quantity of blood under the microscope. A drop of whole, unclotted blood is spread evenly on a glass slide. It is then stained with reagents that enhance the visualization of the cellular components. The count of red and white blood cells, the percentages of the white blood cells present, and the concentration of platelets in the blood are taken.

NONCELLULAR COMPONENTS OF THE BLOOD

Enormous amounts of information can be obtained by examining the cellular components of blood, but even more information is available by measuring the various hormones, minerals, enzymes, and fat levels carried in the blood. These tests are done on the blood serum. A blood sample is most often drawn in the morning after an eight-to-twelve hour overnight fast. It is important to be fasting at the time the blood sample is drawn, as food or drink can alter some of the components that are measured. However, the blood-cholesterol level can be measured in the nonfasting state as a screening technique, but most physicians do prefer that all the tests be done after an overnight fast.

A tube of blood is taken from the arm and allowed to clot. Since cellular components are measured from an unclotted sample, often two tubes of blood are taken, one that will not clot, and one that will. After the blood has been allowed to clot, it is centrifuged rapidly, allowing the clotted blood to descend to the bottom of the tube, leaving what is known as serum.

Blood tests as a whole can be used either to "screen" for disease that is present or to predict impending disease that is not yet present. In modern medicine we routinely use tests to screen for disease but are only recently beginning to use the blood test as a predictor.

Take the example of the average man who has a heart attack. The first changes that occur in him can be found in the blood. His diet and lifestyle cause alteration in the total cholesterol, triglyceride, HDL cholesterol, and uric-acid levels in the blood (see chapter 2). These levels normally, and initially, are very low and safe, and do not stimulate the atherosclerotic deposit of fat and cholesterol in the blood that cuts off flow, bringing on a heart attack. However, for years before a heart attack occurs, the elevation of these factors in the blood is quite evident. Only recently has the elevation of these risk factors stimulated any activity from physicians to reduce them, thus reducing the risks of that first heart attack.

Certain laboratory tests are so commonly done that commercial laboratories have automated machines capable of doing a series of tests, sometimes twenty, at one time. This is certainly high technology, as many of the tests require different mechanisms for evaluation. For instance, the measure of the sodium and potassium level in the blood utilizes an electrical current passed through an electrode that attracts and measures only sodium, or only potassium. Other tests, such as those for enzymes, including AST (SGOT) and ALT (SGPT), discussed later, add reagents or substances to a small sample, shine a light through the sample and assess the concentration of the enzyme by the color produced. The automatic analyzer, from a small sample of serum, allocates enough serum for each test as it passes along an assembly line of technological innovation.

Accurate and rapid testing is so common in modern medicine that hundreds of tests on the blood can be reported to the physician in the hospital within minutes of drawing the blood. Generally, a physician in his office can receive the results of an extensive laboratory panel within twenty-four hours.

The next chapter explains the laboratory panel usually used at the Whitaker Wellness Institute. It is also a laboratory panel that can usually be obtained in any part of this country. These are not all of the tests that can be used on blood chemistry, but an enormous amount of information about health and potential disease can be gained from them.

Each test will be described, giving the American cultural range (which is often considered "normal") for the test, the optimal average, and an explanation as to why the American range may or may *not* be the healthy optimal. In many cases, the American range and the healthy optimal are not the same. If we didn't make the distinction between the typical and the optimal, the test would not be valuable for predicting an onrushing disease since so many diseases—high blood pressure, diabetes, atherosclerosis, etc.—are prevalent among Americans.

It is not the purpose of this book to turn you into your own doctor. The adage that the man who functions as his own lawyer has a fool for a client holds for he who acts as his own physician.

However, you do need to have some understanding of the blood tests generally done if you are going to work with your physician to improve your health and use the blood tests to measure that progress. The next chapter discusses the most common tests from the standpoint of how they can be used to predict problems down the line, and how either diet, exercise, or nutritional supplements can change them.

——— 2 ———

Understanding Laboratory Test Reports

As every patient knows, doctors are dependent upon laboratory tests to refine their diagnoses and to point to problems that may not be evident by either the medical history or physical evaluation.

Although careful medical history will tell the physician a great deal, laboratory tests are the key to pointing out imbalances in the system that are not readily apparent. A routine physical examination offers only a fraction of the amount of information that can be gleaned from laboratory tests of the various functioning components of the body. Ideally, both should be used, thereby maintaining a close doctor-patient relationship while utilizing laboratory tests to the best advantage.

We are just now coming to grips with the impact of laboratory tests as a predictor and indicator of degenerative disease. Unfortunately, most physicians today don't educate their patients about the importance of both positive and negative findings in their tests. However, if you know what to look for in your laboratory tests, you can keep tabs on your system and catch problems early enough to do something about them.

USING TESTS AS AN EARLY-WARNING SYSTEM

We've all had friends or acquaintances who have come down with specific symptoms of disease—stomach pain, chest pain, severe headache and the like—and were admitted to the hospital to undergo "tests." When symptoms, such as a pain or altered function in an individual, arise, a variety of tests are used to determine what is wrong.

Many of the same tests, particularly tests on the blood, can and should be used before any indication of disease is manifest. In this way, the blood tests act as an early-warning system, alerting both the physician and the individual of an "impending" problem.

Using blood tests on a healthy individual is similar to warning indicators in an automobile or airplane. Long before the automobile makes an abnormal sound or loses power, an indicator will warn the driver that the oil level is low, the battery is not recharging, or that the gas tank is almost empty. The more sophisticated the machine, the more sophisticated are the warning indicators. As any mechanic will tell you, it is far less expensive and desirable to add oil to an automobile than it is to repair or replace an engine that has suffered the ravages and destruction of running without adequate lubrication.

UNITS OF MEASUREMENT

Each test is reported to the physician as a numerical number followed by units of measurement. Here are the units that are used and what they mean.

mg% or **mg/dL** (deciliter, which means 100 cubic centimeters, or one in a liter)—This unit is the number of milligrams of the substance that is found in 100 milliliters (one deciliter) of blood. It is commonly used for substances such as glucose, creatinine, cholesterol, urea, and triglycerides, and is simply the measure of the weight of the substance contained in that volume of blood.

gm% or **gm/dL**—The number of grams per 100 cubic centimeters is the measurement for substances which are quite plentiful in the blood, such as the amount of protein, albumin, and globulin.

meq/L—Stands for milliequivalents per 1,000 cubic centimeters (a liter) of blood.

Many substances, such as sodium, potassium, chloride, and magnesium, combine with other substances to form different compounds. For instance a single atom of sodium combines with a single atom of chloride to form the molecule (any substance made of two or more atoms), sodium chloride. A single atom of potassium, like sodium, combines with a single atom of chloride to form another salt, potassium chloride. However, a single atom of magnesium combines with *two* atoms of chloride to form magnesium chloride.

28

Though these substances have different weights, the units of measurement in the blood are milliequivalents, which reflects their combining properties. For instance, 10 milliequivalents of sodium weighs more than 10 milliequivalents of potassium, but their combining properties, milliequivalents, is more important than their weight, so it is the measurement that is used.

U/L—Units per liter are usually used to measure the activity, and thus the amount, of an enzyme circulating in the blood. Enzymes characteristically cause a known substance to react without themselves changing. For instance, enzyme X, when mixed with substance A, produces one gram of substance B. A unit is an arbitrary measurement set up by the lab. For instance, one unit of enzyme X may be the amount of enzyme required to turn one gram of substance A into substance B. Therefore, if the amount of enzyme X circulating in one liter of blood is capable of converting 20 grams of substance A into 20 grams of substance B, the reading would be 20 units per liter.

Since a unit of enzyme activity is an arbitrary measurement, there may be several such measurements used by the various laboratories. Therefore, the normal value for that laboratory for an enzyme measurement will be reflected on the report sheet and may be an entirely different unit system than that reported by another lab. This should not cause a problem, as elevations above normal or average will be reflected regardless of the unit system used.

mcg/mL, ng/mL, pg/mL—These are units of measurement smaller than a milligram that occur in the blood per milliliter of blood. They are used to report concentrations of certain hormones and end products of metabolism in which minute amounts in the blood are important.

COMMON TESTS DONE ON BLOOD SERUM

The following are the most common tests done on the blood and also some of the most valuable. As mentioned above, the average and optimal ranges are identical for many tests, but in this country, where diet and lifestyle create changes in large numbers of people that bring on disease, the average reading may be indicative of an impending health problem.

It is very important to know which test in the routine blood chemistry has "averages" in this country that are different from the optimal level, thus heralding a problem. In addition, it is important to know which tests in the blood have average levels which are identical to optimal levels. In these cases, any variation represents a problem that may not be related to our general lifestyle at all.

TEST	AVERAGE RANGES IN U.S.	OPTIMAL RANGES
Glucose	70–115 mg.%	65–100 mg.%
BUN	10–25 mg.%	8–20 mg.%
Creatinine	.7–1.4 mg.%	.7–1.4 mg.%
BUN: Creatinine Ratio	10–30	10–20
E - Alkaline Phosphatase	30–125 U/L	30–125 U/L
N ALT (SGPT)	0–30 U/L	0–30 U/L
Z - AST (SGOT)	0–34 U/L	0–34 U/L
Y GGPT	4–65 U/L	4–65 U/L
E LDH	100–225 U/L	100–225 U/L
S -		
Total Bilinbin	0–1.3 mg.%	0–1.3 mg.%
Indirect Bilinbin	0–1.0 mg.%	0–1.0 mg.%
Direct Bilinbin	0–1.3 mg.%	0–1.3 mg.%
Calcium	9.0–11.0 mg.%	9.0–11.0 mg.%
Phosphorus	2.6–4.5 mg.%	2.6–4.5 mg.%
Sodium	137–147 meg/L	137–147 meg/L
Potassium	3.8–5.4 meg/L	4.2–5.4 meg/L
Chloride	94–110 meg/L	94–110 meg/L
Magnesium	1.3–2.5 meg/L	1.7–2.5 meg/L
Carbon Dioxide (CO_2)	22–31 meg/L	22–31 meg/L
Uric Acid	2.5–8.0 mg.%	2.5–6.0 mg.%
Triglycerides	50–200 mg.%	50–115 mg.%
Total Cholesterol	150–300 mg.%	under 200 mg.%
HDL cholesterol	30–85 mg.%	over 55 mg.%
LDL cholesterol	60–180 mg.%	under 145 mg.%
VLDL cholesterol	10–40 mg.%	under 40 mg.%
cholesterol: HDL Ratio	3.43–9.55	3.43 or lower
Total Protein	6.4–8.5 gm/dL	3.43 or lower
Albumin	3.5–5.0 gm/dL	3.43 or lower
Globulin	1.4–3.9 gm/dL	3.43 or lower
A/G Ratio	.9–3.6	3.43 or lower

Glucose

Glucose, as most know, is sugar. It is the primary fuel of the body, and most other carbohydrates or simple sugars are converted into glucose before the cell utilizes them.

The blood-glucose level is the primary test for diabetes mellitus. When this test is made it is important for the individual to have fasted for 12 hours, because even normal people will have a blood glucose reading in the 120s to 130s a few hours after eating.

The blood-glucose level is maintained by the interaction of insulin with the body. Therefore, alterations in the blood-glucose level reflect alterations either in insulin production or in the body's response to insulin.

Insulin is like a key that opens the cell door, allowing glucose to leave the blood and enter the cell, where it can be used as energy. Without insulin, or if the body is insensitive to insulin (which we will discuss later), the glucose in the blood is unable to enter the cell, and the blood level of glucose elevates.

Insulin is produced in the pancreas and is released into the blood in response to elevations of glucose. For instance, after eating breakfast, the blood-glucose level begins to rise in response to food intake. This stimulates the pancreas to release insulin, which ideally allows the glucose in the blood to enter the cell, keeping the blood-glucose level within a healthy range.

DIABETES Diabetes is characterized by an excessive level of glucose in the blood, both before and after eating. It occurs in two forms: type one, commonly referred to as insulin-dependent diabetes, and type two, referred to as non-insulin-dependent diabetes. Both forms of diabetes will cause an elevation of blood glucose, but it is important to differentiate the two.

Type-one diabetes is the more severe but certainly less frequent form of diabetes. It results from the inability of the pancreas to produce sufficient insulin. Usually the cells of the pancreas that produce insulin have been damaged or destroyed by viruses or even the body's own immune system, and insulin production simply doesn't occur. Without insulin, the blood-sugar level begins to rise, and diabetes becomes manifest. This form of diabetes, the most severe form, fortunately accounts for only 10 percent of men and women in this country who are diagnosed as diabetics.

Since the problem with this form of diabetes is insulin deficiency, insulin therapy is essential. However, the amount of insulin necessary can often be reduced by a diet and exercise regimen, which, as we shall see below, renders the body much more sensitive to insulin, whether it is produced by the body or injected with a syringe.

Type-two diabetes occurs because the body loses its sensitivity to the insulin that is produced in the pancreas. This is the less severe form of diabetes, and by far the more prevalent, accounting for 90 percent of those who have a diabetic condition. The body's insensitivity to insulin is primarily the result of our sedentary lifestyle, obesity, and high-fat diet.

Excessive amounts of fat in the blood render the insulin insensitive, as if

31

it was plugging up the keyholes in the cells, not allowing insulin to open the cell door.

Obesity and lack of exercise have the same effect upon the body's sensitivity to insulin. In many diabetics, the pancreas may indeed be producing excessive amounts of insulin that simply doesn't work because of loss of body sensitivity.

The treatment for this form of diabetes should not rely on insulin therapy because insulin deficiency is not the problem. The ideal treatment for type-two diabetes (also called non-insulin-dependent) should revolve around low-fat nutrition, weight loss, and exercise, which addresses the problem.

HYPOGLYCEMIA Occasionally, the blood level will reflect very low levels of glucose. In someone who is taking insulin injections, an abnormally low glucose means either too much insulin or not enough food.

True hypoglycemia (the term used to delineate abnormally low blood-glucose levels) is rare in men or women not taking insulin. When it does occur, it generally indicates an insulinoma, a tumor in the pancreas that produces excessive amounts of insulin. This condition must be treated by surgical removal of the tumor.

Occasionally, after a high sugar meal, the body will overshoot in its production of insulin in its attempts to keep the blood sugar from going too high, and the blood sugar will drop below normal. In the 1970s, *functional* or *reactive hypoglycemia* became a fad disease. Numerous books were written on this condition, and almost every manifestation was blamed on functional hypoglycemia. In reality, this functional hypoglycemia is much less common than was believed. Generally, there are other explanations for the symptoms that were commonly ascribed to hypoglycemia fifteen years ago.

Bun

The BUN stands for blood urea nitrogen which is a protein-breakdown product and is a test of the function of the kidney. Protein that is not utilized by the body is generally broken down into urea, creatinine, and uric acid. This breakdown of protein occurs throughout the body, primarily in the liver, but is eliminated by the kidney.

The kidney is continually filtering out these protein-breakdown products, and excreting them in the urine. That is the primary function of the kidney. Slight elevations of the BUN could simply indicate a large protein intake, which will increase protein-breakdown waste products. Another cause for elevation of the BUN is dehydration, or reduced amount of fluid in the body tissues and blood. When the body is dehydrated, the filtering action of the kidney slows down, causing the BUN to elevate. In individuals who drink large amounts of water, which increases the filtering action of the kidney, the BUN levels can be flushed to low levels.

In addition, when the protein content of the diet is reduced, the BUN will characteristically fall. A reduced protein intake is healthy in many respects and certainly takes the stress off the kidney by reducing its workload. Therefore, the optimal range of the BUN is slightly lower than the average range found in American culture, primarily because of the excessive protein consumed by Americans.

Creatinine

Creatinine is another protein-breakdown product found in the bloodstream that is filtered and eliminated by the kidney. Creatinine is primarily a breakdown product of muscle. The levels of creatinine found circulating in the blood are not dependent upon the amount of protein found in the diet or the amount of fluid intake. When the kidney is damaged, losing its ability to filter blood, both the creatinine and the BUN level will rise. However, since the creatinine level in the blood is less altered by protein intake and fluid, it represents a more accurate measurement of kidney function than the BUN.

There are many reasons for kidney dysfunction, and two of the most common are diabetes and high blood pressure. In fact, diabetes is the most common reason for total kidney failure.

BUN:Creatinine Ratio

The BUN:creatinine ratio is a ratio (and therefore has no units of measurement) of the values for BUN and creatinine. It is another index of kidney function and is important because it eliminates the fluctuating characteristics of BUN. As the BUN falls with a healthier, lower-protein diet, the creatinine will generally stay the same, and the ratio will decrease. Therefore the optimal kidney-function levels will be low to below normal BUN, normal creatinine, and a low-normal BUN:creatinine ratio.

Enzymes

Enzymes are catalysts that allow metabolic sequences to progress in an orderly manner. For instance, let us assume that the body needs a certain amount of substance D. D is produced from the original raw product A that is present in food. In order to produce D, A must be converted to B, which must be converted to C, which is converted to D, the body's required substance. Each conversion requires an enzyme, which the body produces. Many enzymes, in order to be functional, require coenzymes, such as Vitamin B_6, zinc, magnesium, thiamine or riboflavin (as discussed in chapter 7). The production pathway for substance D would look like this:

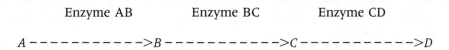

One group of enzymes is called the transaminases and includes AST (SGOT), ALT (SGPT), and GGTP. These enzymes remove nitrogen from protein molecules in the process of protein degradation. They are found in all the cells of the body, but large concentrations of these enzymes are characteristically found in the liver. Therefore, diseases of the liver that destroy liver cells result in substantial increases of these transaminase enzymes in the bloodstream.

Hepatitis, which is the active and acute destruction of liver cells either by a virus or a drug, will often result in a thousandfold increase of the transaminase enzymes. In patients who have had a heart attack, there is likewise a release of transaminase enzymes that can be measured over several days. The degree of elevation of enzymes that are found specifically in heart muscle are helpful in diagnosing whether actual heart damage has occurred, and if so, how much.

There are hundreds of enzymes that can be measured in the blood. Severe malnutrition or vitamin or mineral deficiency will result in a reduction of the production of certain enzymes. In this country, however, severe vitamin and mineral deficiency is rare, but "subclinical" deficiency of vitamins and minerals may occur. Such a condition will not result in an abnormal blood level of enzymes because the enzymes characteristically concentrate and function inside of the cell, not in the blood.

Enzymes are routinely measured, as they indicate the presence of cellular damage. In men or women who are suffering from a combination of several diseases, such as diabetes, heart disease, high blood pressure, obesity, and/or gout, there is often a slight to moderate elevation of the enzymes. The body is loaded with enzyme functions, but only certain enzymes in the blood are frequently measured.

ALKALINE PHOSPHATASE This enzyme is characteristically elevated when there is damage to either the bone or liver. In children, however, alkaline phosphatase is normally high compared to an adult, and is an indication of growth. Likewise, in adults who are "mending" a broken bone, the alkaline phosphatase level is characteristically elevated, as this enzyme is necessary for the normal healing of bone.

TRANSAMINASE ENZYMES: ALT (SGPT), AST (SGOT), and GGTP. These transaminase enzymes are characteristically elevated with liver damage, heart damage, or any other significant tissue damage. The higher elevation, the more the damage. In patients who have suffered heart attacks, transaminases that are specific to heart-muscle damage are measured.

LDH The final enzyme that is characteristically used as a part of a laboratory panel is LDH. This enzyme is present in heart, lung, liver, and muscle tissue. It is elevated with either a heart attack, liver damage, or a pulmonary embolus, which damages lung tissue. It can also be elevated with significant bruising of the muscle, or in men or women who exercise vigorously on a regular basis.

The routine tracking of blood-enzyme levels is important to rule out damage to various organs of the body that may result from disease.

Total, Direct, and Indirect Bilirubin

The measurement of the bilirubin level assesses the ability of the liver to remove the breakdown products of red blood-cell destruction. After its life span of about 120 days, the red blood cell is taken to the liver or the spleen and broken down. The iron from the red blood cell is saved and incorporated into hemoglobin, the essential protein of red blood cells necessary for oxygen transportation. When the red blood cell is broken down, part of the hemoglobin molecule, a biopigment called bilirubin, is released and must be excreted.

Before it can be eliminated from the body, however, it is "conjugated" by the liver into a more water-soluble form, then excreted by the liver via the bile ducts into the intestinal tract and ultimately out of the body in the stool.

If either form of bilirubin is significantly elevated in the blood, the skin and the whites of the eyes become "jaundiced" with this yellowish pigment. Jaundice conditions have been known for centuries.

The laboratory is able to differentiate the two forms of bilirubin, the indirect (water-insoluble), a by-product of the breakdown of red blood cells, and the direct (conjugated and therefore water-soluble), which is produced by the liver. It is important to know the difference for the following reasons.

If there is an increase in production of bilirubin because of rapid blood-cell breakdown, then the level of indirect (unconjugated) elevates and overwhelms the liver's ability to conjugate the bilirubin and excrete it. On the other hand, if the bile ducts of the liver are blocked (as with a bile stone plug) then the level of direct (conjugated) bilirubin increases in the blood.

If there is significant liver damage, as from chronic hepatitis or cirrhosis, then both the indirect and direct forms of bilirubin are elevated. This is why the measurement of total bilirubin is significant.

Diet has very little to do with elevated bilirubin levels. However, excessive ingestion of vitamin A or its analogue beta-carotene can cause a yellowish pigmentation of the skin and whites of the eyes that can appear to be jaundice but isn't. This yellow pigmentation from excessive beta-carotene is harmless and will disappear when the dietary excesses are stopped. Excessive intake of vitamin A, however, will cause liver damage and damage to other organs as well. One should be careful not to take more than 10,000 units of vitamin A per day.

Calcium

The measurement of calcium in the blood is an indicator of the competency of the body's systems to maintain the optimal blood level of calcium. Contrary to popular belief, the calcium level in the blood is *not* an indicator of the adequacy of calcium in the diet. It is important to understand that you can have a very normal blood-calcium level and still lose a lot of calcium from your bones, developing osteoporosis, which can cripple you in later years.

Calcium is essential to optimal health. It is the most common mineral found in our skeletal system and is necessary for the maintenance of the strength of bones and teeth. Calcium is also essential in numerous metabolic reactions, for normal nerve conduction and muscle contraction, and in maintenance of the normal rhythm of the heart.

The blood level of calcium is maintained rigidly between the levels of 9.0 and 11.0 milligrams per cubic centimeter. The blood calcium is very sensitive to hormonal and metabolic changes. When there is either elevation or reduction in the blood-calcium level, then a significant hormonal or metabolic change has occurred.

The most common reason for elevation of the blood-calcium level is hyperparathyroidism. The parathyroid glands, which are small islands of glandular tissue located within the thyroid gland (hence their name), are primarily responsible for maintaining the blood-calcium level within rigid boundaries. A tumor of the parathyroid gland results in excessive production of parathyroid hormone. This hormone will cause the blood-calcium level to elevate.

Additional reasons for elevated calcium levels are malignancy, sarcoidosis (a disease that manifests itself like an infection, even though an infectious agent cannot be found), excessive vitamin D intoxication (usually the dose must exceed 100,000 units a day for several months before this occurs), and insufficiency of the adrenal glands.

Low calcium levels are found with hypo- or inadequate parathyroid hormone production, or failure of the kidneys from any cause.

Diet has relatively little to do with the blood-calcium level in most men and women. This is because the blood-calcium level is maintained within such rigid boundaries by hormonal factors. What is important with respect to bone strength is *calcium balance*. For instance, an individual may ingest 700 milligrams of calcium per day, yet lose 750 milligrams in the urine with a net negative balance of 50 milligrams per day. This additional 50 milligrams of calcium loss comes from the bone. Another individual may ingest 700 milligrams of calcium per day and lose only 650 milligrams of calcium in the urine, with 50 milligrams of calcium deposited into the bone. In both individuals the blood-calcium level will likely be completely normal. It is only calcium balance that is significantly different.

Only at very low levels of calcium intake (200 to 300 milligrams per day) is there negative calcium balance, with more calcium lost in the urine than taken in the food. Most Americans consume approximately 400 to 1,000 milligrams of calcium daily in their food, which is more than enough to maintain calcium balance. In short, we are getting enough calcium.

Then why do we have such severe osteoporosis in the elderly?

The answer is protein. The American diet is excessive in protein. As discussed above, protein must be broken down into urea, creatinine, and uric acid, and excreted in the urine. These breakdown products create an acid condition in the blood, so with a high protein load, the blood becomes acid, and calcium is leached from the bone to act as a buffer. This calcium is then filtered out of the blood by the kidney and excreted in the urine along with the protein-breakdown products. Therefore, excessive protein throws the body into negative calcium balance. All the while the blood-calcium level remains normal. Numerous studies have shown that countries with high-calcium and high-protein diets have significant osteoporosis, while people in countries with low-calcium, low-protein diets maintain the strength of bones and teeth throughout their lives.

Therefore, do not be lulled into a false sense of security about the future strength of your bones simply because you maintain a normal calcium level in your blood.

Phosphorus

Phosphorus is in dynamic equilibrium with calcium and will go in the opposite direction of blood-calcium-level changes. If the blood level of calcium goes up, the phosphorus level goes down and vice versa. Diet doesn't specifically affect the blood level of phosphorus, but a high-animal-protein diet, which is high in phosphorus, causes a negative calcium balance.

Sodium, Potassium, Chloride, and Magnesium

These minerals are called electrolytes and are maintained in strict balance in the blood. Their balance and interaction are necessary for the normal transmission of nerve impulses, muscle contraction, and heart rhythm.

Sodium carries a single positive charge and exists in high concentrations in the blood, as opposed to inside the cell. If you were to eat a high-salt diet, you would have high blood pressure, but the blood sodium would *not* elevate. Any increased intake of sodium would draw more fluid into the blood system to dilute the sodium, keeping it at the normal level, but increasing the amount of fluid in the body, and, thus, the blood pressure. This increased fluid is often experienced as edema and is the reason for "tight rings" and swollen ankles experienced by many after eating movie-house popcorn.

The blood-sodium level *will* elevate with severe dehydration or abnormally increased steroid-hormone production by the adrenal gland. The sodium level will fall with excessive water intake, kidney failure, or inadequate production of steroid hormones by the adrenal gland.

Potassium, like sodium, carries a positive charge. It is in low concentration in the blood and in high concentration inside the cell. The most common abnormality of potassium reported on laboratory screens is an elevation. However, this usually results from the process of drawing blood. If the red blood cells are ruptured when the blood sample is drawn, the potassium, which is in very high concentration inside the cells, is spilled into the serum. Also, if the serum is allowed to "sit" on the red-blood-cell clot after the blood sample has been centrifuged, then potassium will leak into the serum and elevate the potassium level. If the potassium is significantly elevated, then a repeat blood test should be done to confirm that this was a laboratory artifact. Artifact means an abnormal value not associated with an abnormal condition of the body, but with a defect in either the way the blood was drawn, processed, or analyzed by the laboratory.

The blood potassium does rise in kidney failure, however, so in these patients an elevated level is significant.

The second most common abnormality of the electrolytes is a depressed potassium level, which is usually associated with diuretic therapy. Many diuretics that are commonly used cause severe potassium depletion unless potassium is put back into the bloodstream with supplements. Potassium depletion can cause dangerous cardiac arrhythmias and muscle cramping.

Diuretics deplete the body of not only potassium, but also magnesium, calcium, chromium, manganese, and zinc. Diuretic therapy should be closely monitored, and should not be utilized unless absolutely necessary. Most of the time, a prudent diet and an exercise program are all that is necessary to lower the blood pressure, but for those who still require medication there are alternatives to diuretic therapy. For many, the use of diuretics constitutes a greater hazard than a completely untreated condition of mild high blood pressure.

Chloride is the negative ion that can combine with sodium, potassium, or magnesium (all positive ions) to create sodium chloride, potassium chloride, and magnesium chloride. In a liquid medium such as the blood, sodium, potassium, and magnesium chlorides disassociate and remain in the liquid.

Only rarely is chloride altered in the blood. Occasionally, excessive vomiting or excessive water drinking can lower the chloride level in the blood, though this is relatively rare. Chloride is elevated in the blood by dehydration or kidney failure. For most conditions that alter the chloride level in the blood, however, other laboratory tests are more specific for diagnosing the condition than the blood-chloride level.

Magnesium is a mineral that is found both within and without the cell and is extremely important in numerous metabolic reactions. It also is necessary to stabilize normal heart rhythm as well as muscle contraction. In patients with both heart disease and diabetes, magnesium levels in both the blood and tissues are found to be depleted.

In patients who have just had a heart attack, the magnesium concentration in the monocytes is found to be significantly lower than normal.

In the diabetic patient the magnesium level in the blood is on the average lower than the optimal level, and in those who suffer with progressive eye damage the magnesium level is even lower. At the Whitaker Wellness Institute, the blood-magnesium level is routinely measured, and magnesium supplementation is often advised for all patients on the nutrition and exercise regimen.

Carbon Dioxide (CO_2)

Carbon dioxide in the blood, which is actually bicarbonate, is the body's primary buffer in helping to maintain a stable pH balance. The pH is a measure of the acidity or alkalinity of the blood. The pH of pure water, which is equally balanced between acid and alkaline, is 7. If the pH measurement drops, the acidity of the solution increases. If the pH increases, the alkalinity of the solution increases. Blood is maintained at a pH of 7.4, slightly alkaline.

When metabolism in the body increases the acid concentration, the acid is absorbed by the carbon dioxide and the level of carbon dioxide begins to drop. If an alkalizing condition develops, such as excessive vomiting, which causes the loss of substantial amounts of HC1 (hydrochloric acid), then the CO_2 level goes up. In both conditions, the fluctuation in the CO_2 level is far greater than the fluctuation of the pH balance, since the CO_2 acts as a buffer, stabilizing the pH.

Acid conditions of the blood can be either metabolic, such as from poorly controlled diabetes, which causes the acid to build up with marked reduction in the CO_2 level, or respiratory, as from inadequate ventilation of the lungs, which is often seen in patients with severe lung disease from cigarette smoking. Aeration of the lungs allows the body to blow off carbon dioxide gas (not the bicarbonate that is also called carbon dioxide), eliminating acid.

An alkaline condition of the blood can likewise be either metabolic, such as from excessive vomiting (see above) or respiratory, as from hyperventilation (excessive breathing), which depletes the body of hydrogen ions by blowing off excess amounts of CO_2 gas.

Uric Acid

Uric acid, like BUN, is a protein-breakdown product. It is important to measure the concentration of uric acid in the blood, because if the level is elevated, the uric acid will migrate out of the blood, into the joints and precipitate into crystals, causing inflammation and arthritis. This is called gout.

The tendency toward elevation in uric-acid levels is often inherited, but a high-protein diet plays a big role as well.

Sometimes the uric-acid level will elevate during a period of weight loss and will fall again once weight has stabilized at a lower level. A diet lower in animal protein but higher in vegetable protein and fiber is helpful in reducing the uric-acid levels. High uric-acid levels are also strongly associated with heart attacks. Like cholesterol, high uric acid serves as an early warning sign of potential atherosclerosis and heart problems, but is not as widely appreciated as the blood-cholesterol level. Therefore, if the uric-acid level in the blood is elevated, even closer attention to the other risk factors of heart disease is important.

Another common reason for uric-acid elevation is diuretic therapy. In fact, the highest uric-acid measurements in the blood are found in patients taking large doses of diuretics, and, in particular, thiazide diuretics. Thiazide diuretics include HydroDIURIL, Dyazide, Hydrochlorothiazide, Moduretic, and Maxzide. When the uric acid is elevated above 8 milligrams per cubic centimeter, it should be treated first with a lower-protein diet, then with uric-acid medications if necessary.

Triglycerides

Triglycerides are neutral fats circulating in the blood. After eating a fatty meal, the triglycerides elevate over the next several hours and coat the red blood cells, causing the red blood cells to clump together, thus reducing the oxygen supply to the cells.

Elevated triglycerides also play an important part in the development of atherosclerosis. A high level of triglycerides decreases the oxygen available to the artery wall, causing subtle damage to the artery lining, opening the door for fat and cholesterol to deposit, build up, and eventually close off the artery. In addition, triglycerides are a part of cholesterol deposits that plug arteries.

The triglyceride level in some cases can elevate to the thousands. When the triglyceride level goes above 300 milligrams per cubic centimeter, the serum of the blood becomes turbid. The higher the level, the more turbid the serum becomes. In extreme cases of triglyceride elevation, the serum begins to take on the consistency of cream.

Factors that elevate the triglyceride level are dietary excesses of fat and sugar, alcohol, lack of exercise, and obesity. Diabetes, alcoholism, and pancreatitis are also associated with elevated triglyceride levels. Extreme elevations of triglycerides can cause acute, painful cases of pancreatitis by clogging the circulation to such an extent that the pancreas releases its powerful digestive enzymes and damages the tissues of the organ. Diuretics and oral contraceptives will also elevate the triglyceride level.

These dangerous fats can be lowered rapidly with the right program. Factors that lower the triglyceride levels are: a low-fat, low-calorie, high-fiber diet; exercise; and weight loss. Fish oil is particularly helpful in cases with marked elevation. The oil of cold-water fish contains eicosapentaenoic acid, an omega-3 fatty acid (discussed in more detail in chapter 4) that rapidly lowers both the triglyceride and cholesterol levels when they are both elevated.

Cholesterol

Blood cholesterol is probably the most important measurement for predicting future heart disease. Cholesterol is not itself a fat; however, since it is attached to fatty carriers in the blood, it is usually discussed along with fats.

Cholesterol is essential to our well-being; we need a certain amount in our bloodstream. It is necessary for production of the sex hormones estrogen and testosterone, as well as the steroid hormones produced in the adrenal gland.

Cholesterol is essential in the production of vitamin D which controls calcium metabolism and protects the skin from ultraviolet light. Cholesterol is produced in the liver and in other cells, where all the cholesterol necessary for its myriad functions is supplied.

It has been estimated that a blood-cholesterol level of 120 milligrams per cubic centimeter is enough for the cholesterol to perform all of its essential functions in the body. Ingestion of cholesterol is never required; therefore, cholesterol is not a "nutrient." The American diet, which is very high in cholesterol, saturated fats, and animal protein, elevates the cholesterol level substantially.

Since the whole country is consuming essentially the same types of food, the average cholesterol level is substantially higher than in countries on a diet oriented toward more vegetable protein. For instance, the cholesterol level in Japan ranges from 120–170, while the cholesterol level in the United States ranges from 150–300, with the average in this country 211.

It is only recently that physicians have become aware that the "average cholesterol level" is far from optimal and is actually indicative of serious heart disease later in life.

THE CHOLESTEROL CARRIERS Just as rubber tires rolling down the highway are always attached to cars or buses, cholesterol molecules traveling in the blood are always attached to a carrier composed of protein and fat. Cholesterol is transported in the blood by three different types of *lipoproteins* (a combination of fat and protein).

The three carriers and their attached cholesterol molecules can be separated and then measured by contrifuging very rapidly (ultracentrifugation) a tube of blood. The different densities or weights of the carriers depend upon the percentage of protein or fat. The *high-density lipoprotein* (HDL) contains the most protein, and therefore is the heaviest, migrating to the bottom of the tube upon centrifugation. The *low-density lipoprotein* (LDL) contains a mixture of fat and protein, is lighter than the HDL, and migrates to the middle of the tube with centrifugation. The *very low-density lipoprotein* (VLDL), made up almost completely of fat with very little protein, is the lightest of the three lipoproteins and therefore stays at the top of the tube after centrifugation.

Another method of separating the three lipoprotein carriers and their cholesterol molecules is by electrophoresis. A drop of serum is placed on a piece of filter paper. An electrical current is passed through the paper, causing the various elements in the blood to migrate across the paper. The HDL, LDL, and VLDL cholesterol carriers migrate at different rates, and thus can be separated and measured.

We will discuss more about the importance of these lipoproteins, but for this section it is enough to say that HDL cholesterol is protective against heart disease, decreases the rate of artery blockage, and can be considered preventive of the complications of atherosclerosis.

LDL cholesterol is the real culprit. It goes into the arteries, blocks circulation, and is responsible for strokes, heart attacks, and other ailments caused by atherosclerosis.

VLDL is also a culprit, but not nearly so dangerous as the LDL cholesterol. Its danger is lessened by its very light, fluffy nature, making it too bulky to attach to the artery. However, it does not prevent atherosclerosis.

CALCULATING LDL AND VLDL CHOLESTEROL Many laboratories will measure only the triglyceride level, the total cholesterol level, and the HDL cholesterol. They will then calculate the VLDL cholesterol as well as the LDL cholesterol.

The first calculation is for VLDL cholesterol. The VLDL fraction of cholesterol is carried in the triglycerides that are circulating in the blood. It has been found the VLDL cholesterol is equal to .2 times the triglyceride fraction, or the triglyceride fraction divided by 5.

With this calculation we now have total cholesterol and HDL cholesterol (which were measured), and the VLDL cholesterol (which was calculated). We can now calculate the LDL cholesterol. The formula for this is: Total cholesterol − HDL − .2 × triglyceride (VLDL) = LDL.

This is a very valuable formula.

CHOLESTEROL:HDL RATIO It has been determined that as the level of the total cholesterol of the blood goes up, the risk of heart disease goes up as well. It has also been determined recently that as the level of the HDL cholesterol goes up in the blood, the risk of heart disease goes down. This is confusing on the surface because both the total cholesterol and the HDL cholesterol are, in fact, cholesterol. The total cholesterol happens to be dangerous (because the majority of total cholesterol is LDL cholesterol), while one fraction of the cholesterol (HDL) is protective.

One way of relating these conflicting factors is to create a ratio between cholesterol and HDL. When the total cholesterol is divided by the HDL, a single number is obtained. If the total cholesterol level stays the same and the HDL fraction increases, the number achieved by the ratio is reduced. As this cholesterol:HDL ratio decreases, the risk of heart disease decreases as well.

For instance, a man with a total-cholesterol level of 220 and an HDL-cholesterol level of 44, would have a cholesterol:HDL ratio (220 divided by 44) of 5.0. This cholesterol:HDL ratio is the average in the country and thus represents the average risk of having a heart attack. Since about 50 percent of American men die from heart disease, it is quite dangerous to walk around with average risk.

Another man has a cholesterol level of 220, but an HDL cholesterol of 65. His cholesterol:HDL ratio (220 divided by 65) equals 3.4. This ratio is consistent with one half the average risk of heart attack. An individual with a cholesterol level of 220, but an HDL cholesterol of 23 has a cholesterol:HDL ratio of 9.5 which is consistent with twice the average risk.

For women the risk of having a fatal heart attack is, overall, about one-tenth that of men. The cholesterol:HDL ratio which is consistent with the average risk of heart attack for women is 4.4, one half average equals 3.3, and twice the average equals 7.1. Women generally have higher HDL cholesterols and lower total cholesterols, so their average ratios are lower than that of men.

OPTIMAL CHOLESTEROL:HDL RATIO Just what is optimal? The answer to this

44

is simply: How much risk do you want to walk around with? What is optimal, therefore, is a judgment by either a physician or an individual. Our personal recommendation is to get your cholesterol:HDL ratio to at least one half the average risk, or 3.4 for men, and 3.3 for women. If it is lower than this, all the better.

Total Protein, Albumin, Globulin, and A/G Ratio

The blood is chock-full of protein, which can be separated into albumin and globulin for a variety of reasons. A molecule of albumin is roughly one half the size of a molecule of globulin.

Albumin is very much involved in transport of a variety of substances throughout the body, including free fatty acids, and many of the electrolytes, such as calcium and magnesium. The albumin level is a rough estimate of the nutritional state; decreased albumin levels in the blood indicate malnutrition. Significant malnutrition can either be primary, resulting from lack of food and essential nutrients, or secondary, as a result of malabsorption, malignancy, or other chronic disease. Primary malnutrition is very rare in the United States, but affects approximately 25 percent of the population in Africa and Asia.

Levels of albumin between 3.0 and 3.5 grams per deciliter, which are indicative of malnutrition, can occur without symptoms. If the albumin level drops below 3.0, then edema, lethargy, bone resorption, and muscle wasting generally occur.

Globulins, as mentioned before, are a major component of the body's immune system. Globulins carry antibodies throughout the system that react to foreign particles. They can be reduced by severe malabsorption, but many chronic diseases often increase their level. Chronic infection, liver disease, and many malignancies are associated with an increased globulin fraction in the blood.

As important as proteins are in transporting nutrients and substances throughout the body and maintaining a humoral (fluid) defense system, an equally important function is the maintenance of the blood volume. Without adequate levels of albumin and globulin, particularly albumin, fluid leaks from the blood into areas around the cells, and an abnormal fluid accumulation (edema) is formed.

A/G RATIO The A/G ratio, or the ratio between albumin and globulin, is normally between .9 and 3.6. It was considered in the past to have some relevance in differentiating protein abnormalities in the blood. However, the understanding of these protein abnormalities and their relationship to various diseases is such that today the A/G ratio is no longer considered significant. It is very important to assess the albumin and globulin as well as the components of them.

PROTEIN ELECTROPHORESIS AND THE IMMUNE SYSTEM An assessment of the globulins in general and the immunoglobulins (those globulins associated with immunity) in particular can be done by protein electrophoresis. A drop of serum is placed on filter paper and then subjected to electrical current causing a migration of the various globulins across the paper. In this manner the specific humoral globulins can be assessed and their percentage of the total globulin calculated.

MEASUREMENT OF INTRACELLULAR MINERALS

Blood tests, helpful as they are, sometimes do not give an accurate picture of what is going on *inside* of the cell. This is particularly true of several minerals whose concentration inside the cell is higher than the concentration in the blood. Even when blood values of these minerals are normal in the blood, the condition inside the cell could be grossly abnormal.

Magnesium and potassium are two minerals whose concentration in the cell is significantly higher than the concentration in the blood. For instance, about 98 percent of the magnesium and about 90 percent of the potassium in the body is contained inside of the cell, with only 2 percent and 10 percent respectively contained in the blood.

Since most of the magnesium and potassium in the body is contained inside of the cells, there could be significant depletion of the body stores of these two minerals long before there is any noticeable change in the blood level. This is often the case in diabetes, high blood pressure, heart disease, and obesity. In addition, until the *cellular depletion* of these two minerals is corrected, these dangerous conditions will not improve.

Therefore, blood values of these minerals can be misleading. In addition, the intracellular *ratios* of these minerals—magnesium to calcium and sodium to potassium—are important and cannot be determined with the blood test.

In the past, intracellular analysis of minerals has been inaccurate. The cells often had to be obtained by invasive techniques, such as a biopsy. In fact, until recently there has been no routine intracellular mineral analysis available to physicians in the office or even in hospitals, where laboratory support is extensive.

But all of that is changing now with the development of a test that is inexpensive, accurate, and can be used by a physician in his office. Before discussing this test, however, let's review some of the changes that occur in the mineral balances within the cells with the onset of various diseases.

There are certain patterns that occur with high blood pressure, heart disease, diabetes, osteoporosis, and cardiac arrhythmia, but in general the pattern that is usually common to all is an *increase* in cellular concentration of *calcium, phosphorus, sodium,* and *chloride,* and a *decrease* in cellular *magnesium* and *potassium.*

All of the minerals are balanced by cellular pumps and metabolic functions, so a shift in one will usually cause a shift to some extent in all of the minerals. For instance, sodium is pumped out of the cell, but potassium is allowed to stay. The calcium concentration inside the cell is determined indirectly by the sodium-potassium pump as well, and its concentration begins to rise when the sodium-potassium pump slows down. Therefore, one of the first indications of a problem would be an increase in the concentration of calcium inside the cell. This is seen in early and chronic stages of heart disease, high blood pressure, and osteoporosis.

Early measurements of the shift in concentration of intracellular calcium is more valuable than the blood level of calcium, since the blood-calcium level generally stays well within normal limits during these intracellular shifts. Reduction of magnesium and potassium is the other side of the coin and will almost always be associated with increased intracellular calcium.

How the Tests Are Done

Recently, Dr. Burton B. Silver, director of research at Spectroscan Corporation in San Bruno, California, developed a novel technique to measure intracellular concentrations of minerals, and the National Aeronautics and Space Administration (NASA) has since used this technique to measure intracellular minerals in several experiments they have conducted on the effect of weightlessness on calcium shifts.

A scraping of the cells in the buccal mucosa (under the tongue) is placed on a microscope slide and prepared with a fixative. These cells are then bombarded with a high-voltage electron beam. Each mineral reacts to the energy of the electron beam in a characteristic manner, and a specific pattern of energy is generated that can be quantified. This energy pattern is then

47

accurately correlated to the various concentrations of calcium, phosphorus, magnesium, sodium, chloride, and potassium in the cell. The units of measurement of this test (which you certainly do not need to remember) are expressed as X-ray intensity, peak/background per unit cell volume, which is abbreviated as EXA units. With one test, the physician can receive information on the concentrations of each mineral inside of the cell as well as their ratios.

Bed Rest, Zero Gravity, and Cellular Calcium

It has long been known that bed rest will stimulate rapid calcium losses from the bone. Our skeletal system requires that it be put under stress with walking or other forms of exercise for maintenance of bone strength caused by calcium remodeling. Bed rest and extremely sedentary living cause the calcium to mobilize out of the bones and then to be excreted in the urine, a possible cause of disuse osteoporosis. What has only recently been appreciated is that when calcium is mobilized from the bone, the *concentration* of calcium inside of the cell *increases*.

Astronauts who spend long periods of time at zero gravity lack the gravitational stress upon the skeleton necessary to maintain bone strength, which is why NASA is very interested in studies that demonstrate early calcium shifts out of the bones and into the cells in response to zero gravity or lack of exercise. NASA commissioned a study on five healthy adult males in which their intracellular minerals were measured before and after twenty-seven days of bed rest in a six-degree head-down position. The result was a significant *increase* in the intracellular content of calcium, which indicated that calcium was being pulled from the bones, and was increasing in the cells.

Cellular Calcium (EXA units)	
Normal range	56–102
Control (before bed rest)	81 plus or minus 14 (normal)
Day 27 bed rest	109 plus or minus 15 (high)

Mineral Shifts and Other Diseases

Using this test, Dr. Silver has demonstrated significant alterations in patients reporting to the emergency room with various conditions. In patients reporting with atrial fibrillation, a sometimes rapid and always irregular heart-

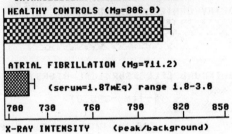

U.S. ARMY EMERGENCY ROOM PATIENTS
INTRACELLULAR MAGNESIUM LEVELS

HEALTHY CONTROLS (Mg=806.0)

ATRIAL FIBRILLATION (Mg=711.2)

(serum=1.87mEq) range 1.8-3.0

700   730   760   790   820   850

X-RAY INTENSITY   (peak/background)

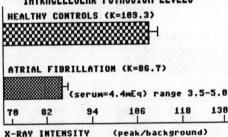

U.S. ARMY EMERGENCY ROOM PATIENTS
INTRACELLULAR POTASSIUM LEVELS

HEALTHY CONTROLS (K=109.3)

ATRIAL FIBRILLATION (K=86.7)

(serum=4.4mEq) range 3.5-5.0

70   82   94   106   118   130

X-RAY INTENSITY   (peak/background)

beat, the *intracellular magnesium* and *potassium* levels were significantly *low* in comparison to healthy controls, but the *blood level* of these two minerals was *within acceptable ranges*. We have already mentioned that magnesium and potassium are crucial for maintaining the normal heart rhythms.

Compared to healthy controls, those patients undergoing bypass surgery for heart disease had significantly lower intracellular magnesium, and significantly higher intracellular calcium and phosphorus. The tests taken on the sublingual cells from the mouth were verified by biopsy samples taken from the atrium of the heart and the aorta.

Those being treated for high blood pressure or other forms of heart disease similarly had low cellular magnesium, yet elevated calcium and phosphorus concentrations.

MAGNESIUM IN SUBLINGUAL SMEARS, ATRIUM AND AORTA (BY-PASS PATIENTS)

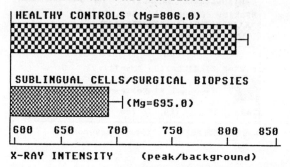

HEALTHY CONTROLS (Mg=806.0)

SUBLINGUAL CELLS/SURGICAL BIOPSIES

(Mg=695.0)

600   650   700   750   800   850

X-RAY INTENSITY   (peak/background)

PHOSPHORUS IN SUBLINGUAL SMEARS, ATRIUM AND AORTA (BY-PASS PATIENTS)

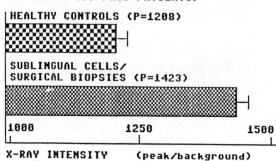

HEALTHY CONTROLS (P=1208)

SUBLINGUAL CELLS/
SURGICAL BIOPSIES (P=1423)

1000   1250   1500

X-RAY INTENSITY   (peak/background)

CALCIUM IN SUBLINGUAL SMEARS, ATRIUM AND AORTA (BY-PASS PATIENTS)

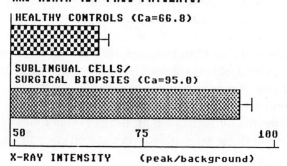

HEALTHY CONTROLS (Ca=66.8)

SUBLINGUAL CELLS/
SURGICAL BIOPSIES (Ca=95.0)

50   75   100

X-RAY INTENSITY   (peak/background)

50

INTRACELLULAR SUBLINGUAL IONS: HYPERTENSIVE/CARDIOVASCULAR DISEASE

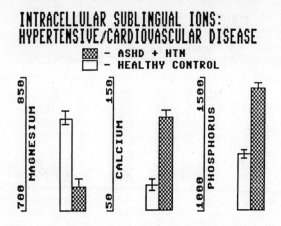

Since these changes in the intracellular minerals occur before and are more significant than the changes in the blood minerals, they represent a very powerful tool in predicting potential problems down the line as well as assessing the value of treatment. It has been shown that exercise will increase intracellular potassium and magnesium levels, and cause a reduction in intracellular calcium and phosphorus.

In addition, treatment with magnesium seems to be more important than treatment with calcium to restore intracellular order. For instance, patients with periodontal disease, before treatment with magnesium, had very low magnesium concentrations, as well as elevated intracellular calcium and phosphorus. After one year of treatment with magnesium, there was a very significant increase in intracellular magnesium, almost approaching normal, as well as a corresponding drop in intracellular calcium and phosphorus. Bone density, as measured by dental X rays, appeared to improve or stabilize, and correlated well with the sublingual intracellular measurements of these minerals.

51

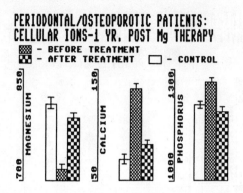

PERIODONTAL/OSTEOPOROTIC PATIENTS:
CELLULAR IONS-1 YR. POST Mg THERAPY
▓ - BEFORE TREATMENT
▒ - AFTER TREATMENT   ☐ - CONTROL

These tests are now routinely done on patients that enter the Whitaker Wellness Institute.

3

Blood Tests as Early Indicators of Interconnecting Disease

Trash newspapers seem to take the "single-bullet" approach to describing the cause and effect of diet on blood and evolving degenerative disease. "If you avoid fat, you'll never have heart disease." "If you eat more carrots, you'll protect yourself from cancer." "If you never eat liver, you'll never be troubled by gout." The list of claims goes on and on. Each statement has a germ of truth in it that has been exaggerated. The solution is not to eliminate one food or to add one food, but rather to follow the broad spectrum of a balanced-nutrient diet that will keep your blood profile in a normal range.

What is needed is a thorough understanding of how we cause our own defeat by ignoring combinations of abnormal blood-test scores that pave the way to one or many forms of degenerative disease. As you will see, lifestyle has a great deal to do with spoiling the health of later years.

There is a link between such health problems as hypertension, atherosclerosis, heart disease, and diabetes. It is not always possible to predict which of these degenerative diseases will appear first, but if certain blood tests continue to be abnormal, sooner or later the body will succumb to the physical breakdowns that have the same poor test scores in common. These include high cholesterol and triglyceride levels, a poor cholesterol:HDL ratio, and high glucose readings.

Another link is between gout, arthritis, and osteoporosis, with *high uric acid count being a basic tipoff that joint disease is on its way.* When the uric acid level in the blood elevates, it deposits in the joints and causes inflammation.

53

It is not always possible to spot osteoporosis potential because calcium is leached out of the bones and may be plentiful in the blood as the bones become more porous and fragile.

A similar link exists between digestive diseases and colon cancer, and is not often spotted by a blood test—diet based on refined foods. The lack of fiber in this kind of diet contributes toward sluggish bowel-transit time, which can cause the formation of diverticulosis (outpouchings along the intestinal wall) and further complications of colon health.

If you are used to eating on the run and grabbing haphazard meals, it is quite possible to develop a blood profile that begins to give warnings of abnormalities. If these are left unchecked, the conditions can worsen, until it is much like a game of Russian roulette—the gun may only be loaded with one bullet, but sooner or later it's going to be fired.

THE HUMAN CONDITION AT BIRTH

The day we were born most of us were in excellent health. Barring any genetic abnormalities, we all weighed about the same, had about the same degree of activity, and, for the most part, ate exactly alike. If we were breast-fed we received food and nutrients that were "specifically planned" to supply all our nutrient needs for that early growth phase, with the correct mixtures of fats, carbohydrates, and proteins. And grow we did. We doubled our weight in six months (imagine doubling your weight in six months now!), we increased the size of our brain by close to 300 percent, and we experienced extremely rapid growth in our bones, muscles, and organs.

A blood sample at age one year or younger is substantially different than that taken at ten years, twenty years, or later in life. The enzyme levels (SGOT, SGPT, LDH, and alkaline phosphatase) are generally 200-400 percent higher than in the adult. This significant increase in enzymes represents the marked enzyme activity of growth.

The blood-fat levels are also substantially lower. It is not unusual for an infant to have a blood-cholesterol level of 65 and a triglyceride level of 50. Many laboratory measurements, such as calcium chloride, CO_2, total protein, and albumin, are roughly comparable to levels found in the adult.

What is interesting about human infants, particularly those that are breast-fed, is that the "variation" in the "variable" laboratory measurements (those that are sensitive to diet and other factors of our lifestyle) vary less than that of the adult. Simply stated, the range of the blood-cholesterol level, triglyceride, blood-sugar level, and uric acid is "tighter" (fluctuates less).

Moreover, the diseases that afflict the infant and pediatric age are caused primarily by infections either with bacteria or viruses. These diseases represent a "right of passage" as the infant adjusts to the rather hostile environment of earth. His immune system is continually challenged with various diseases, programming itself for an effective defense the next time around.

Additional diseases of the infant and pediatric group are congenital, such as cystic fibrosis, birth defects, and muscular dystrophy. In short, the pediatric age group does not generally suffer from diseases brought on by "lifestyle" unless that lifestyle happens to be particularly unhealthy.

When children begin to eat the adult foods of the family, their blood values quickly alter, particularly the cholesterol and triglyceride levels, which are rapidly altered by diet. However, children rarely develop heart disease, arthritis, or the other degenerative diseases so common in the adult population. Children and even adolescents seem to have a reserve of strength that protects them. These blood alterations, however, set the stage for deterioration later in life, so routine blood screening of children on at least a yearly basis, is appropriate.

THE OLDER CHILD

During adolescence, all blood values are similar to adult values, with the ranges reflecting the differences in diet preferences. The teen years begin to set the stage for problems in adult life as lifestyle patterns are solidified. However, the most significant problem for most during this time is simply the stress of being a teenager in modern society.

The early to mid-twenties are certainly more significant for blood chemistry than the teen years and should be the time of active intervention to avoid problems later on. During the mid-twenties, exercise for many is dramatically reduced. Throughout high school and the college years, most participate in some form of regular physical activity, whether in organized team sports or physical education. In early adult life the stimulus for continuation of physical activity rests solely on the shoulders of the individual. In fact, the responsibilities and stresses of this period generally reduce physical activity and stimulate poor nutrition.

A blood panel will invariably chronicle these changes. The fasting blood-sugar level will begin to rise, even if it stays within normal limits, going from 80 milligrams per cubic centimeter to perhaps 105 milligrams per cubic centimeter. The uric-acid level will rise, but only slightly. Big changes occur in those measurements that are most sensitive to diet and exercise—total cholesterol, HDL, LDL, VLDL, and cholesterol:HDL ratio. There is a tendency for the total cholesterol and LDL fractions to elevate, as well as the triglyceride level.

At this time, physicians should be very aggressive with their young patients, impressing upon them the importance of good diet and exercise to avoid disability in the later years. Unfortunately, almost without exception, men and women in their twenties continually get a false stamp of good health regardless of blood warnings that could be addressed.

TWO CASE HISTORIES

Let's imagine two scenarios. Bill S. is a good example. During high school and college he was extremely active, competing in track during high school, and for four years on the rowing team in college. His diet was extremely high in carbohydrates, as he had learned by experience that carbohydrates supplied him with the energy he needed for training and competition. His blood cholesterol level ranged from 140 to 165, and his triglyceride level was very low, measuring only 65. His blood pressure was 118/70, and he weighed 165 pounds on a six-foot frame.

Bill graduated from college and went to work for an advertising agency. He was working ten to twelve hours per day, and his exercise fell to zero. His diet deteriorated to fast foods and restaurant fare. Within six months his weight had ballooned to 195 pounds, his cholesterol shot up to 218, his triglyceride increased to 200, and his blood pressure shot up to 140/85.

All of his measurements were still within "normal" range based upon current practice, so no alarm bells sounded for either his doctor or himself. However, the course was set, and unless he significantly reverted back to his healthier way of living in some way, he was likely scheduled for a health calamity in his fifties or sixties.

His experience can be contrasted with Henry A., who was similar to him in activities and blood measurements up until both graduated from college. Henry also went to work for an advertising agency, worked the same hours, but for some reason decided to make exercise a priority and continued to eat healthy, low-fat foods. It took a little more effort and time, but six months out of college he had gained only seven pounds, his blood-cholesterol level measured 170, triglyceride 110, and blood pressure 120/85.

Let's Jump Ahead

At forty-eight years of age, let's check in on Bill and Henry and examine what has happened to their blood profile over the twenty-seven years since graduation from college. By the time Bill and Henry reached forty-eight they had dramatically separated themselves with respect to their laboratory profile, state of health, and, most particularly, warning signals for impending disease. Bill's complete laboratory panel is found on the left, Henry's is found on the right and the current accepted ranges for the laboratory used are found in the middle.

	BILL	*AMERICAN AVERAGES* NORM	HENRY
Glucose	>119	70–115 mg/dl	87
BUN	>26	10–25 mg/dL	10
Creatinine	1.4	0.7–1.4 mg/dL	1.0
BUN: Creatinine ratio	14.4	10–30 mg/dL	10
Uric Acid	>8.1	2.5–8.0 mg/dL	4.6
Calcium	9.7	9.0–11.0 mg/dL	9.7
Phosphorus	4.0	2.6–4.5 mg/dL	3.5
Alkaline Phosphatase	118	30–125 U/L	46
LDH	>130	100–225 U/L	70
ALT (SGPT)	>41	0–30 U/L	20
AST (SGOT)	>36	0–30 U/L	14
Bilirubin Total	1.4	0–1.3 mg/dL	1.0
Total Protein	8.4	6.4–8.5 gm/dL	6.9
Albumin	4.8	3.5–5.0 gm/dL	4.2
Globulin	3.2	1.4–3.9 gm/dL	2.7
Cholesterol	281	150–300 mg/dL	165
HDL	45	30–85 mg/dL	55
LDL	171	60–180 mg/dL	93
VLDL	65	10–40 mg/dL	17
Cholesterol: HDL ratio	6.2	3.43–9.55 mg/dL	3.0
Triglyceride	325	50–200 mg/dL	87
Sodium	139	137–147 meql/L	139
Potassium	3.9	3.8–5.4 meql/L	4.9
Chloride	94	94–110 meg/L	99
CO_2	26	22–31 meg/L	26
Magnesium	1.3	1.3–2.5 meg/L	2.1
Hemoglobin	16	14–16 mg/dL	14
Hematocrit	47	37–47%	42

Chart continued on page 58.

White Blood Cell	9.0	4.8–10.8	4.4
Polymorphonuclear Neutrophils	70%	42–47%	60%
Lymphocytes	20	20–51	30
Monocytes	5	1.7–9.3	5
Eosinophils	3	2–4	3
Basophils	2	2–4	2

Let's examine Bill's panel:

• His fasting glucose is up moderately. This indicates that the high-fat diet, lack of exercise, and obesity have destroyed his ability to handle carbohydrates. He now has mild diabetes.

• His BUN is up slightly, but his creatinine is normal. This increase of BUN certainly reflects the large amount of meat and protein in his diet.

• His uric acid is also elevated because of the high-protein intake, and no one would be surprised if Bill had an attack of gouty arthritis in the very near future.

• His calcium level is normal, as is his phosphorus level.

• Bill's enzymes are slightly elevated. The degree of elevation is not high. This represents mild cell damage throughout the system (the cause of the severe derangement that has occurred in his metabolism over the past twenty-eight years).

• His bilirubin is normal, no significant liver damage has occurred

• His total protein is not out of range, it is at the high end of that range primarily because of his high normal albumin level. Bill eats a lot of protein and is "overnourished."

• There are major and alarming changes in his blood-fat measurements, which are the most sensitive to lifestyle changes and which are also the most predictive of significant disease. His cholesterol level is now 280, HDL 45, LDL 171, VLDL 65, cholesterol:HDL ratio 6.2. This profile of the blood fats is consistent with rapid buildup of cholesterol deposits in the arteries that lead to heart attacks and strokes.

• Potassium and magnesium levels are slightly depressed. By this time Bill is already hypertensive and has been started on a thiazide diuretic as a first treatment. He is taking a potassium supplement, but not enough, as his potassium level is in the low-normal range. In addition, his magnesium level has dropped as well. Low magnesium and potassium levels are dangerous, as this condition indicates instability in the heart rhythm. Also, relative minor changes in the blood levels of potassium and magnesium usually represent major disruptions in the balance of these two minerals inside and outside of the cell.

• An examination of his blood count shows a high-normal hemoglobin and hematocrit. A high-protein diet stimulates red-blood-cell production, giving him more red blood cells than are needed to supply oxygen adequately. This elevation in red blood cells simply makes the blood more viscous and increases the likelihood of an abnormal clot. Several studies have shown that as the red-blood-cell mass increases above the level necessary to carry oxygen, there is an increase in frequency of both stroke and heart attack.

• His white-blood-cell count is at the high-normal range. It has just recently been realized that a high white-blood-cell count, even though within the average range, is significantly associated with an increased risk of heart disease. In a recent study, published in the *Journal of the American Medical Association* of May 1, 1987, it was found that those with white-blood-cell counts in the high-normal range (greater than 9,000 per cmm) had four times the risk of heart attack or stroke compared to those with white blood cell counts in the low-normal range (less than 6,000 per cmm). Most of the risk is associated with polymorphonuclear elevation. Seventy percent of Bill's white blood cells are polys.

The reason for this increased risk appears to be the function of white blood cells in the progression of atherosclerosis. There are two ways the white blood cell can facilitate the progression of artery damage.

First, they play a surprisingly important part in the flow characteristics of the blood even though they make up less than one percent of all the blood cells. The white blood cell is larger than the red blood cell and therefore can block the circulation at the level of the capillary. It takes only a few white blood cells to plug up a capillary, and when this happens the white blood cell may damage the capillary by releasing oxidants, causing swelling and even more blockage.

Second, they adhere to the areas of damage in the endothelial cell barrier of large arteries and release toxic substances that perpetuate this damage, accelerating the atherosclerotic process.

It is important to realize that the elevations of the white blood counts that indicate a fourfold increase in risk of heart disease are still within what is generally accepted as "normal," which is another reason why the laboratory test should be used to aid in predicting problems down the line.

If we now look at the entire picture presented to us by Bill's complete laboratory panel, we see that in every area that is observed, it appears that his internal metabolic systems are near the breaking point. He is on the verge of full-blown type-two, non-insulin-dependent diabetes, gouty arthritis, high blood pressure (for which he is now already taking a diuretic), severe atherosclerosis (putting him at risk of having both a heart attack and a stroke), and likely cancer of the colon or prostate, which we shall see is intimately associated with the high-protein, high-cholesterol diet of the American culture. Yet, other than medication for his mild high blood pressure, he has received no significant medical attention for what is going on in his body.

At this time he had best seek out a hospital and try to reserve a bed (perhaps at a reduced rate), because he's going to need it.

Henry, on the other hand, reached forty-eight still carrying his optimal weight with a blood pressure of 120 over 80, a commitment to regular exercise, and the discipline necessary to choose high-complex-carbohydrate, low-fat, low-protein food. His blood panel has optimal levels *in all areas.* There is no indication of *any* of the chronic diseases that most Americans suffer and die from. Just as Bill's complete laboratory panel indicates complete breakdown in several areas, which will become manifest as one of several diseases, Henry's laboratory panel indicates metabolic systems that are running smoothly, quietly, efficiently, and are in optimal condition.

At this stage of the game, Bill could significantly alter his lifestyle, and dramatic changes would predictably occur. All of the indicators of impending disease could be reduced. But at this point Bill is very close to the edge. Once you fall off and begin to have heart attacks, diabetes, or strokes as complications of atherosclerosis and high blood pressure, or significant deterioration of the joints from arthritis, it becomes more difficult to regain health.

A NEW PICTURE FOR DISEASE

What is needed is a different set of beliefs about our major killing and debilitating diseases. For most people suffering ill health, the disease, be it cancer, heart disease, diabetes, high blood pressure, osteoporosis, or obesity, is not a genetic accident, an act of God, transmitted by bacteria or virus, or bad luck of the draw. Rather, the disease is a predictable, multifaceted response to the way we live.

Our beliefs about disease do not connect them to our daily lives, so that as we get older we are ever more likely to develop one or several problems that have been brewing in our systems for years. The gradual alteration and deterioration of the blood panels, examined from a preventive standpoint, herald the onslaught of our major problems. Unfortunately, Western medicine has treated alteration in these blood changes as "age-related." This is just not true. Blood-cholesterol level, blood pressure, weight, and other alterations in the laboratory and physical measurements are factors more of lifestyle than of age. But because they occur so frequently, age is a convenient scapegoat.

The key to optimal health is not taking blood tests, but living in a way that insures health. The rest of the book gives you all you need to do that: diet information, how to start an exercise program, and a reasonable nutritional supplement program.

What follows is the map for optimal health that everyone should be following, but especially those whose blood tests put them at high risk for disease. The blood tests are like the signpost along the road that help each person keep on track for health.

Ready to get started?

Well, here is what to do and why.

—— 4 ——

What Blood Tests Can Reveal About Your Food Habits

One of the keys to controlling blood chemistry is controlling your food intake. There is a direct correlation between blood-test results and your food choices. Changing your approach to food can reverse your blood warnings. It's amazing how the body will respond to being treated like the high-powered fuel consumer it is. Excess fat floating in the blood in the form of cholesterol and triglyceride takes a nosedive when you fail to provide a high-fat, high-sugar diet. Hypertension (high blood pressure) studies show that when sodium is drastically reduced in the diet, pressure falls to normal ranges. Calcium added to the diet in the form of skim-milk products adds protein as well as bone-building and repairing capabilities, besides giving reported protection to the heart and blood system by lowering the blood pressure.

Your medical destiny can show up in your blood many years before trouble strikes. Changing your food habits can reverse abnormal blood-test scores and keep them in a normal range for the rest of your life. It's not a matter of going on a special diet for one particular problem, but rather of going on a well-balanced regimen to prevent all problems.

If you are showing a high blood-cholesterol level and/or a high triglyceride level, it reveals that you are courting potential problems with heart and artery disease. Add to that a high-blood-pressure report, and you can count on dealing with hypertension as well. If your blood sugar is high, you are inviting adult-onset diabetes. And if you are obese, you may be involved with all of these when you could and should be enjoying a good life.

The common denominator of these diseases is that they are caused by your fork. They involve eating excess fat, excess protein, excess sugar, and excess salt. In addition, if you eat refined foods (white flour, white rice, white bread) most of the time, you are going to miss the B vitamins and fiber found in whole grains. Additional fiber is needed from fruit and vegetable sources to speed up the digestive process and prevent colon cancer.

LABORATORY TESTS ALTERED BY DIET

The following is a list of the routine laboratory tests done by physicians that are *generally* altered by our nutrition. In addition, these tests have the ability to predict disease in the future, which we will expand upon further.

Glucose (fasting) is generally increased by high-fat, high-sugar, high-calorie nutrition, obesity, and lack of exercise. It is reduced by lower-fat, lower-calorie nutrition, weight loss, and exercise, and is the initial predictor for diabetes.

Urea nitrogen is generally increased to the upper limits of normal by high-protein nutrition. It is substantially decreased, sometimes by 50 percent, with a lower protein intake. It will elevate substantially with kidney dysfunction.

Uric acid increases with high-protein, high-calorie nutrition and obesity, and decreases with vegetable proteins, lower calories, and weight loss. There is a transient increase during weight loss, which falls after weight loss has been established. High levels of uric acid are indicative of potential arthritis from gout and heart disease.

Total protein and albumin are generally higher as a result of a meat-based diet. Shifting to lower-fat nutrition will cause a mild drop in both total protein and albumin, but still within healthy ranges. These factors are not particularly predictive of oncoming disease.

Cholesterol (HDL, LDL, VLDL) is highly sensitive to nutrition. It increases with saturated fat, cholesterol and animal proteins in the diet, and substantially decreases with low-saturated fat, vegetable proteins, and fiber. Total cholesterol is highly predictive of oncoming heart disease.

Triglyceride is very responsive to nutrition, though not as responsive as cholesterol. Triglycerides are increased with high-fat intakes, sugar, and inadequate fiber, as well as obesity and lack of exercise. Triglycerides are lowered with lower-fat nutrition, lower sugar intake, higher fiber, exercise, and weight loss. Triglycerides are predictive of cardiovascular disease (though not as much as cholesterol), diabetes, and possibly cancer.

Calcium in the blood is rigidly controlled by hormones usually irrespective of dietary fluctuations. However, it is listed in this group as being affected by diet because the "calcium balance" of the body is so strongly associated with protein intake. A persistent negative calcium balance is the reason for osteoporosis in later years.

Magnesium is weakly altered by diet and by decreased intake of magnesium. Blood levels are still maintained rigidly. Low levels are weakly predictive of impending heart disease and possibly diabetes.

LABORATORY TESTS NOT ALTERED BY DIET

Enzymes (alkaline phosphatase, LDH, ALT, AST) are indicative of disease already present, but are not particularly helpful in predicting disease. However, in people suffering from a variety of diseased conditions, these enzymes, which are indicators of cellular damage, are often elevatd.

Sodium, potassium, chloride, and carbon dioxide are not generally altered by diet, nor are abnormalities in their level predictive of oncoming disease. Abnormalities generally reflect a condition that is occurring at the time.

The important thing about the blood tests is that they generally indicate what your food habits are and how much exercise you are getting. They reflect the state of your general health, and as your habits change, they affect your health for better or worse.

Usually the first sign of a health disaster is heralded by these changes long before you begin to "feel bad."

FAT

All fat has about 100 calories per level tablespoon. This is true whether the fat is from butter, margarine, shortening, vegetable oil, or animal fat. Some people continue to believe that margarine has less calories than butter. Not true. Or they think that vegetable oil can be consumed in unlimited amounts because it has no cholesterol. While it may be a more desirable choice, it is still a fat and should be controlled in the diet. Still others trim all of the fat around their meat but eat large portions without regard for the invisible fat that is marbleized throughout the meat. Fat has a way of adding up calories because it has about 9 calories per gram, while protein and carbohydrates have about 4 calories per gram.

To put this information into perspective, suppose you are considering buying a product that gives you nutrition information stating that there are 200 calories per serving and the fat content is 9 grams per serving. Multiply the

9 grams by 9 calories per gram and you quickly find out that 81 of the 200 calories are composed of fat. The knowledgeable choice is then up to you.

Such arithmetic is important when you are analyzing your food intake. For instance, the majority of Americans now eat a diet in which 45 percent of the total calories they consume is in fat. That means, if they eat 2,000 calories a day, 900 of those calories are taken in as fat. A healthier proportion is to eat 20 percent fat in your diet, so that only 400 calories of the 2,000 would be attributable to fat.

But even that kind of restriction isn't enough; the kind of fat you choose is just as important as the amount you eat because fat falls into several categories. You should be able to recognize the sources of saturated fat, poly-unsaturated fat, and monounsaturated fat whether you prepare your own food or it is served to you.

Saturated Fat

Saturated fat contains cholesterol. It comes from animal sources, such as meat, poultry skin, butter, and cream. This is the kind of fat that can clog your arteries and cause atherosclerosis as it calcifies. It is very similar to a thick rust buildup in plumbing pipes, except in humans the plumbing pipes turn out to be the arteries that need to be wide open so that red blood cells can carry a maximum of oxygen to every capillary and arteriole throughout the body. Saturated fat is almost impossible to avoid, but it can be done if you do the following:

• It is preferable not to eat red meat. If you do, eat only 3 to 4 ounces of lean meat at a sitting. Trim it well before cooking. Learn to bake, broil, braise, and boil.

• Remove all visible fat from poultry. Never eat the skin. Use cooking techniques that skip the browning-in-oil step. Avoid fried chicken like the plague—if it is served to you, be sure to peel it down to the meat.

• Use only low-fat or nonfat dairy products. Learn to use buttermilk in salad dressings, yogurt in place of cream, and sapsago cheese instead of high-butterfat cheese such as Brie. Other low-fat hard cheeses are gammelost, German hand cheese, and farmer cheese. One-percent cottage cheese and skim-milk ricotta cheese may also be used in cooking to produce a high-calcium, low-fat dish.

• Egg yolks are almost solid fat. Each yolk contains 274 milligrams of cholesterol. They are not recommended. Whites are solid protein with zero cholesterol. Since it is advisable to limit your cholesterol intake to only 100 milligrams or less each day, you can readily see that it is extremely important to learn to cook with just the whites whenever possible. When baking, choose recipes with just egg whites and unsaturated oil. Egg-substitute products are inadvisable, as they are extremely high in sodium, which defeats the purpose for those who are dealing with potential heart disease.

• Vegetable shortening has been hydrogenated to make it solid. In so doing, the unsaturated oil becomes more saturated. Learn how to bake with vegetable oil instead.

• Lard is animal fat. That means it is a solid saturated fat. Avoid it!

Polyunsaturated Fat

Unsaturated fat is vegetable fat, such as corn oil, safflower oil, and sunflower oil. It does not contain cholesterol as long as it is used in its liquid form. However, it does have 100 calories per tablespoon and can add up very quickly if you do not control your use of it.

Palm oil and coconut oil are the exceptions to the rule. They are more saturated and therefore have some cholesterol content. This is important to know because these oils are often listed on labels of fabricated foods. Limit your intake of them.

Monounsaturated Fat

Monounsaturated oil has become one of the hottest nutritional items ever since monounsaturates were proved effective in reducing harmful LDL (low-density lipoprotein) cholesterol while protecting helpful HDL (high-density lipoprotein) cholesterol in the blood.

Olive oil, long a staple of Mediterranean cultures, has by far the highest concentration of monounsaturates—72.3 percent of its fat by volume. Peanut oil is next with a 48.1 percent concentration of monounsaturates. Most other vegetable oils are polyunsaturates, with the ability to reduce both LDL and HDL cholesterol. But, if possible, it's best to preserve HDL, which helps protect against artery disease, while lowering LDL to normal levels.

For this reason, while you are limiting the amount of total fat in the diet, if you need a bit of oil for salad dressing or for sautéing, olive oil or peanut oil is a wise choice. The oils from all plant sources are referred to as omega-6 oils, whether they are polyunsaturated or monounsaturated.

COMPOSITION OF VEGETABLE OILS

OIL	%POLYUNSATURATES	%SATURATES
Safflower	75	9
Corn	59	13
Soybean	58	14
Sesame	42	14
Peanut	32	17
Palm	9	49
Olive	8	14

Source: U.S. Department of Agriculture

The Omega-3 Factor

A source of a highly polyunsaturated oil is the omega-3 factor found in fish oils. Omega-3 fatty acids have been defined by Dr. Roger Illingworth, associate professor of medicine and biochemistry at Oregon Health Sciences University, as linolenic acid. Dr. Illingworth explained to an American Heart Association conference that while linolenic acid is manufactured exclusively by plants, when it is eaten by animals it is metabolized into omega-3. When fish eat plankton, a part-plant, part-marine substance, this conversion takes place.

The oils from all fish contain omega-3, but fish oil found in cold-water fish seems to have the most. For this reason, it is wise to include several fish meals from so-called fatty fish. Some of these fish are bluefish, herring, mackerel, salmon, sturgeon, trout, and tuna.

Research is ongoing with the omega-3 factor. For now, it is known that this factor not only reduces triglyceride levels in the blood but also may reduce clotting by inhibiting platelet clumping in the blood.

Do the Proportions of Fat Intake Matter?

Yes. Health statistics show that the American diet of 45 percent fat calories is a killer habit.

The American Heart Association recently lowered its recommendation from 30 to 35 percent fat calories in the diet to less than 30 percent. A growing number of health experts have concluded that it is now considered wise to limit all types of fat to 20 percent of your caloric intake if you want to reduce your blood-cholesterol level. It is best to get the majority of the fat in your diet from vegetable sources.

Reducing Fat in Your Diet

By now you know that fat surrounds meat and should be trimmed away, lurks under poultry skin, abounds in cheese and other whole-milk products, and provides the taste found in most sauces and creamed soups. But are you aware of how much fat may be hidden in other foods?

- Of the 900 calories found in a pastry pie shell, there are 60 grams of fat. Multiply 60 by 9 calories per gram of fat and you find that the fat content of the pie shell is 540 of the 900 calories. Three-fifths of the pie shell is fat.
- Of the 65 calories found in two tablespoons of cheese sauce, there are 5 grams of fat, which, multiplied by 9 calories per gram, equals 45 calories of fat. About two-thirds of the sauce is fat.
- Of the 255 calories found in one cup of ice cream, 14 grams of fat × 9 = 126 calories of fat. About half of the ice cream is fat.
- Of the 350 calories found in a one-twelfth slice of yellow cake with icing, 13 grams of fat × 9 = 117 calories of fat. About one-third of the cake is fat.
- Of the 275 calories found in a Danish pastry, 15 grams of fat × 9 = 135 calories of fat. About half of the pastry is fat.
- Of the 190 calories found in 2 tablespoons of peanut butter, 16 grams of fat × 9 = 144 calories of fat. About three-fourths of the peanut butter is fat.
- Of the 160 calories found in a glass of whole milk, 7 grams of fat × 9 = 63 calories of fat. About one-third of the milk is fat.
- Of the 50 calories found in a chocolate-chip cookie, 2 grams of fat × 9 = 18 calories of fat. About one-third of the cookie is fat.

Getting the fat out of your food supply is going to take concentrated effort, and nothing beats reading labels. The largest percentage of ingredients are listed first, with the rest in descending order. Some labels now list grams of fat. You now know the formula of finding out how much of the calorie intake is in fat; multiply the grams of fat by 9 and compare it to the number of calories per serving. Since no more than 20 percent of your diet should be fat, there should be no more than 20 fat calories per each 100 total calories you eat.

Watch out for new products that claim to have no cholesterol. They may be high in fat, even though the product has no animal fat, which always contains cholesterol. While foods from vegetable sources do not contain cholesterol, they may not be low in saturated fat. For instance, nondairy creamers, most of which are made from coconut or palm oil, may have no dairy cholesterol but will still be high in saturated-fat content. A better choice would be low-fat or skim milk, nonfat dried milk, or evaporated skim milk.

Some frozen desserts are based on tofu, leading you to believe that they are low in fat. Not so. Some are high in polyunsaturated vegetable oil rather than butterfat, and you'd be better off choosing a scoop of ice milk or soft ice cream. The best choice would be fruit ices, fruit-juice bars, or low-fat frozen yogurt. Even better are some of the poached and pureed fresh-fruit recipes in the dessert section of this book.

PROTEIN

Although protein is vital to the growth and maintenance of all body tissues, we tend to eat more than necessary in the modern diet. All we need is between 12 percent and 15 percent of our calories in protein. The recommended daily allowance, as determined by the National Research Council Food and Nutrition Board, is between 44 and 56 grams of protein for healthy adults. This can usually be accomplished by eating two servings of 3 or 4 ounces of poultry (skinless), fish (not fried), or skim-milk dairy products a day. When combined with grains at the same meal, a higher amount of protein is absorbable. Postoperative patients generally need extra protein for healing.

Excess protein puts stress on the kidneys and can produce high uric acid, leading to symptoms of gout. Excess protein is never stored; the body eliminates it daily through the kidneys. In other words, you must eat protein every day to maintain the body's repair system and hormone system, but even excess amounts only stress and damage the body.

A protein deficiency will affect growth and tissue development. In adults, this can produce weakness, susceptibility to infection, and poor healing ability. In children, protein deficiency can lead to a disease known as kwashiorkor, which affects growth and tissue development to such an extreme that the child can have stunted mental and physical growth, swelling of joints, and loss of hair pigmentation.

To know if you are getting enough but not too much protein, once again turn to arithmetic. If you have one serving of fish containing 34 grams of protein and one serving of white-meat chicken at 30 grams, you have already consumed 64 grams of protein. In place of one of the animal-protein servings, try to substitute two servings of vegetable protein (totaling 15 grams), which gives you 45 or 49 grams, which is not above the recommended range.

Depending on your weight, you are quite close to having enough protein for the day.

High-Quality Vegetable Sources of Protein

Some vegetable sources of protein, such as beans and lentils, are higher in protein than many meat products. It was commonly believed in the past that great effort was needed to "balance" the vegetable proteins to form "complete" protein. Most scientists now realize that a diversified vegetable diet will supply more than adequate protein for all our needs.

There are really no reasons to eat animal protein, but regular ingestion of fish or small amounts of chicken or turkey are certainly acceptable. Fish provides the most protein (34 grams) per four-ounce serving of boneless and skinless flesh. Freshwater fish are a good source of minerals such as copper, iron, magnesium, and phosphorus. Saltwater fish, including all forms of shellfish, provide sources of cobalt, fluorine, and iodine. At one time it was advised to avoid fatty fishes, but now that we know about the role of the omega-3 factor in lowering the triglycerides in the blood while thinning the blood to avoid abnormal clots, it is wise to plan to have several fatty-fish meals each week. Be sure to prepare fish without fat of any kind. Poach it, broil it, bake it—but never ever fry it!

Egg whites and dairy products are another kind of animal protein. Each egg white can provide about 7 grams of protein. Learn how to make beaten egg white omelets from the recipe section in this book to take advantage of this complete and reasonably priced source of protein.

While whole milk should be avoided because about 50 percent of its calories come from fat, skim milk has no fat at all. One cup of skim milk provides about 8 grams of protein and about 300 grams of calcium. All dairy products also supply vitamins B_1, B_2, B_6, and B_{12}. Comparison of the content of protein in cheeses shows that one ounce of low-fat cottage cheese provides about 4 grams of protein, while one ounce of Cheddar cheese provides about 7 grams.

THE CONFUSION ABOUT CARBOHYDRATES

In years gone by, "starch" was a nutritional dirty word. No more. In fact, the current thinking of nutritional scientists is to use starchy food—pasta, potatoes, rice, and bread—to replace the high-fat, high-protein killer diet. Starches don't make you fat—excess fat and sugar do!

Starches are part of the menu offerings of complex carbohydrates. Other complex carbohydrates are vegetables and fruits. All have fiber content that enables the bowel to function with regularity, and all have a wide variety of vitamins and minerals that contribute to well-being.

Complex carbohydrates are metabolized and enter the blood slowly, enabling your blood-sugar level to maintain a regulated balance. By contrast, simple carbohydrates—sugar, syrup, fructose, and honey—are metabolized swiftly since they are already refined before you eat them. They can send your blood-sugar levels on a roller coaster and wreak havoc with your health if taken in large amounts.

When you limit your fat intake to 20 percent of the calories you consume, and protein intake to 12 to 15 percent, then you have 65 to 68 percent of the total calories left over for complex carbohydrates. That figure can represent a lot of very fine eating—with extra servings of grains, vegetables, and fruits.

It's best, however, to choose whole grains such as wheat bran, oat bran, brown rice, kasha (buckwheat groats, a genus related to the rhubarb family), rye flour, and unbleached flour. These ingredients are rich in B-complex vitamins, which are heavily involved in brain chemistry.

When you choose refined flour, even if it is enriched by the manufacturer, some of the vitamins and minerals are missing. In fact, they are in nature's proportion as found in whole-grain foods.

You also have to eat a wide variety of vegetables and fruits. It's time to educate your taste buds to experience the fascinating flavors that occur naturally in fresh vegetables and fruits. Each is bursting with certain gifts of vitamins and minerals. When you eat a wide variety of them throughout the day, you can't miss creating a pool of nutrients your body needs.

While all vegetables are rich in vitamin C, the dark yellow and dark green vegetables also offer good sources of vitamin A in the form of cancer-protective beta-carotene.

Citrus fruits are also rich in vitamin C, and in addition provide a good supply of potassium. Other fruits provide a wide variety of minerals and fiber.

Most important, when you eat more grains, fresh vegetables, and fruits, you are eating more fiber as well. Fiber is that plant material that is not absorbed and does not add any nutrients to the diet. What it does do is bulk up the colon so that you will have regular bowel movements without resorting to laxatives. This in turn is the most protective measure you can take against colon cancer. Eat fiber as if your life depends on it. It does!

SUGAR

Is it all right to eat some sugar since it is a simple carbohydrate? you may ask. That all depends on how much sugar you generally consume in a day. A teaspoon of sugar has 15 calories. That doesn't sound like much, but in fact it can add up. If you stir two teaspoons of sugar into each cup of coffee and are in the habit of consuming eight cups a day, you can easily slip 240 calories into your diet that have no nutritive value.

Brown sugar and honey, while simple carbohydrates, are absorbed a little more slowly into the bloodstream than refined white sugar. Some people find that date sugar, available in health-food stores, has more sweetening power and causes you to use less.

It's important to read food labels to be able to identify different types of simple carbohydrates. You might find a listing for sucrose, glucose, galactose, fructose, maltose, dextrose, lactose, and other "-ose"-ending products, as well as corn syrup and maple syrup. They can add up to a lot of sugar calories.

Watch out for flavored yogurts that have heavy, sugary jams added to them. Most packaged convenience foods are heavily laden with a variety of sugars.

Sugar is a natural ingredient but, by the time it is stripped of its husk and refined of its natural molasses, little nutrition is left. It wouldn't matter too much if you limited yourself to the ten pounds per person per year that people consumed at the turn of the century and before. Now that total of refined sugar per person has increased to over 120 pounds a year. It's hidden in baked goods, condiments, canned soups, prepared mixes, and soda pop. It totals up to a lot of wasted calories and poor nutritional intake.

ARTIFICIAL SWEETENERS

There's bad news about them, too. According to a report from the Division of Nutritional Sciences, Cornell University, ingredients such as sorbitol and mannitol have the same number of calories per teaspoon as sucrose or any other sugar. Although chemically they are not sugars, about twice as much of these two ingredients are needed to equal the sweetness of sucrose.

Any "sugarless" product that is not low or reduced in calories must be labeled as such or contain a statement that indicates a usefulness other than weight control. For instance, some labels of sugarless bubblegum state: "Does not promote tooth decay—not noncaloric." Research with laboratory animals has indicated that both sorbitol and mannitol are less cavity-promoting than glucose, sucrose, or fructose.

The Cornell report also calls attention to diet beverages that contain two types of sweeteners—one that provides calories and one that does not. This means that "diet beverages" are not necessarily calorie-free. They cite low-calorie cranberry-juice cocktail as one example that contains filtered water, cranberry juice, high-fructose corn syrup, vitamin C, and calcium saccharin. Both high-fructose corn syrup and calcium saccharin contribute to the sweetness of this beverage. The high-fructose corn syrup is a type of sugar that adds calories, while the calcium saccharin sweetens without adding calories.

Because this beverage contains both types of sweeteners it must be labeled: "Contains sugars. Not for use by diabetics without advice of a physician." Such diet beverages must contain 50 percent fewer calories than their regular counterparts and provide no more than 6 calories per fluid ounce. Some people who must control their intake of sugar fail to realize that fructose, honey, corn syrup, and brown sugar are converted quickly to glucose, as is refined white sugar.

Sorbitol can present other problems besides adding unwanted calories to meals of unsuspecting consumers. According to a report by N. K. Jain, M.D., in the *American Journal of Gastroenterology*, some patients displayed a sorbitol intolerance that masqueraded as irritable-bowel syndrome. At present the FDA requires that if a product provides more than 50 grams of sorbitol over the period of one day, the following words must be on the label: "Excess consumption may have a laxative effect." Whether you reach the 50 grams or not, it is wise to remember that sorbitol can cause unexplained gas, bloating, or even diarrhea in some people.

Foods can often be prepared with no sugar or sweetener at all. Or, it is possible occasionally to use frozen concentrated apple juice in small amounts as a natural sweetener. Many of the recipes in this book will show you how to do it!

SALT

A salt-free diet is probably one of the least understood terms in modern times. We have become so used to "the great salt lick" of modern food manufacturing that our taste buds have forgotten the marvelous flavors of real food. The good news is that it takes just about three weeks to retrain your taste buds to savor a less salty menu, and after a while you will not want to eat the "salty" food you are eating now.

Some foods have natural sodium in their content, such as beef, poultry, fish, vegetables, and grains. Interestingly, the sodium intake you get naturally in a well-varied menu equals about 2,000 to 2,500 milligrams of sodium a day—just about the amount you need to keep the very special sodium/potassium cellular balance system functioning well. However, modern consumers have been boosted to take in over four times that much by adding salt to cooking and neglecting to consider how much sodium has been added to prefabricated foods. Just one teaspoon of salt added to a pot of soup will add 2,300 milligrams of sodium to it. No wonder there is an epidemic of hypertension among adults who eat this way!

Salt appears on food labels under various names, most commonly sodium chloride. But if you read further the label may list other sodiums as well: monosodium glutamate, sodium bicarbonate, brine, disodium phosphate, sodium alginate, sodium benzoate, sodium hydroxide, sodium propionate, and sodium sulfite.

These hidden sodiums can add up to a lot of sodium content that you don't realize is there when you buy a commercial product. Most labels should list a total amount of sodium. If you know that you are getting as much as you need (unless you are a perspiring athlete) by eating natural unsalted food, why should you add thousands of milligrams of sodium to wreck the balance of your intercellular system?

Far from proposing that you should now eat tasteless food, we suggest you give up the salt shaker and the entire battery of "sodiums" and learn how to season your food with herbs and spices. There's no great mystery to using oregano, dillweed, rosemary, thyme, and basil to pep up your cooking. As a matter of fact, you will become a better cook. You will also learn when to use a bay leaf, how to perk up flavor with whole cloves or grated lemon rind, and when to add onion, garlic, and green peppers to give tangy tastes. All of the recipes in this book are salt-free delicious food.

Now that we have shown you how your food habits affect your blood tests and your health, we need to show you how to make the right changes. The next chapter reveals how to get your diet in shape. Do that, and you get in shape. Now let's get rid of those bad habits and see what happens to your blood tests as well as to your health.

Remember, the whole purpose of this book is to help you make the changes that will make you healthier.

5

Getting Excess Protein, Fat, Sugar, and Sodium out of Your Bloodstream

While some signs of degenerative disease are silent, giving no warnings until the disease is a fait accompli, others are readily apparent in the blood. A habit of continually eating an imbalanced diet, with excesses of protein, salt, simple carbohydrates, and/or fat can give blood warnings that should be heeded.

For instance, an excess of protein can cause a high uric-acid blood level, which if unchecked can lead to gout and arthritis. High protein intake can also play havoc with the potassium/sodium intercellular balance system, affecting blood pressure and heart health.

An excess of simple carbohydrates (sugar, honey, syrup), often hidden in your fabricated food supply, in ice cream, and in desserts, can cause high triglyceride levels in the blood. The sugar is frequently combined with excess fat, causing problems with glucose levels as well. Ignoring low or high glucose test scores can lead to hypoglycemia or diabetes.

An excess of fat in the diet can lead to a myriad of blood warnings, including high cholesterol, high triglycerides, high uric acid, and abnormal glucose levels. Such test scores are warnings of atherosclerosis, heart disease, gout, arthritis, and diabetes.

All are controllable by better management of your dietary intake. Here's what you need to know about abnormal blood levels caused by excesses of food you eat.

THE EFFECT OF EXCESS PROTEIN

All of your life you've been told to eat meat and drink milk because you need a lot of protein to stay healthy and strong. Yet, copious amounts of protein, found in meat, eggs, and whole-milk dairy products, are loaded with saturated animal fat (cholesterol) that plugs up the arteries and causes heart attacks, diabetes, obesity, gout, and some forms of cancer. Lean meat, more skinless poultry, more fish meals, and using only low-fat dairy products can improve the situation.

Even with these precautions, it's necessary to limit your intake of protein. Carbohydrates and fats can be stored in the body in fat-storage cells, but not protein. Fats and carbohydrates contain carbon, hydrogen, and oxygen atoms that make up their molecules, which the body readily converts to energy. Protein is never used for energy, except during starvation. Even then the body's protein must first be converted into glucose before it can be burned as energy.

Proteins, like carbohydrates and fats, contain carbon, hydrogen, and oxygen, but also contain nitrogen, sulphur, and phosphorus. The body cannot store these elements, so they must be evacuated. These three elements cause problems when excessive protein is ingested.

In order for the body to rid itself of excess protein, the protein molecules first must be broken down into urea, creatinine, and uric acid by the liver. These are then transported to the kidney and filtered from the blood to be eliminated in the urine. When excessive amounts of protein are ingested, the liver is stressed, creating an acid condition in the blood. Acidic blood is a major cause of osteoporosis and puts stress on the kidney, which must filter and excrete these products.

Keep in mind that the problem of excess protein occurs primarily in cultures that consume a large amount of protein from animal sources. It would be difficult to obtain excessive protein from vegetable sources, as vegetable protein is less concentrated than animal protein. Vegetable protein is also accompanied by carbohydrates and fiber, which are absent in animal protein foods but provide a satiety value and a sense of fullness that discourages overconsumption. Therefore, when vegetable protein is eaten to meet your caloric needs, there is little reason to worry about excess.

Kidney Disease and Excess Protein

In 1986 the *Medical Tribune* reported that the relationship between protein and renal disease was the subject of a multicenter, five-year, National Institutes of Health–funded study that would follow 1,000 patients with established cases of kidney disease. The study was instigated by the finding that a low-protein diet could delay or even halt the progression of renal disease. Writing in the *New England Journal of Medicine* (Vol. 307: 652, 1982), Dr. N. Brenner states, ''There appears to be a fundamental mismatch between the design of the human kidney and the amounts of protein consumed in the Western diet.'' Forcing your kidneys to filter and excrete 50 to 100 grams of unnecessary protein daily is like driving your car at 8,000 RPM when it was designed to be driven at 3,500.

Diabetes and high blood pressure are two degenerative diseases that significantly damage the kidney. When the kidney fails, the protein-breakdown products rapidly accumulate in the blood and death is not far away. The dialysis machine is used to filter the blood of these breakdown products. This artificial-kidney machine is a lifesaver, but the stresses of kidney dialysis are large, and the quality of life is diminished. Diabetes is the number-one cause of complete kidney failure and the reason thousands of patients now require kidney dialysis.

In patients with diabetes and high blood pressure, the kidneys fail gradually. The blood-creatinine level, as discussed in chapter 2, is the most sensitive measurement of kidney function. Any elevation of the creatinine indicates that kidney damage has occurred. In fact, there must be a 50-percent reduction in kidney function before the creatinine is elevated at all.

As damage to the kidneys continues, the creatinine continues to elevate, indicating further loss of kidney function. It is generally believed by most doctors that when the kidney begins to fail, it will gradually progress to complete failure and that nothing can be done to stop this progression. However, recent studies have shown that if diabetic and hypertensive patients with early kidney damage are put on a low-protein diet, the progressive nature of kidney failure can be stopped, even reversed in some cases. The low-protein diet advocated contains about 35 to 50 grams of protein a day, exactly what has been determined to be the quantity of protein necessary for good health in the adult.

Immunity and Excess Protein

It has long been known that reducing the amount of protein in the diet will significantly enhance the immune system of the body. Why this is so has not been determined, but as early as May 31, 1971, it was reported in the *Journal of the American Medical Association* that since reduction of the protein intake enhanced the strength of the immune system, patients with viral, protozoal, or fungal infections may one day be treated by reducing their protein intake. Since that time, not much experimentation has been done to determine how powerful protein reduction would be in the treatment of disease, but obviously, reduction of protein intake down to the level that covers our needs is warranted for everybody.

Gout and Excess Protein

In addition to urea and creatinine, protein is broken down into uric acid, which is also excreted by the kidneys. If the uric-acid level is increased, it begins to crystallize in the joints of the body, causing gouty arthritis. The protein foods that are most likely to cause an elevation of the uric-acid level are those foods that are rich in DNA and RNA proteins found in the nucleus of the cells. These foods would include organ meats, dried legumes, anchovies, sardines, herring, mackerel, scallops, wild game, goose, tongue, meat broths, meat extracts, gravy, and yeast.

THE EFFECT OF EXCESS FAT

As mentioned in the previous chapter, the body requires a 20-percent intake of fat calories to keep it functioning at normal levels. The current general intake of over 40 percent nationwide has contributed greatly to almost epidemic proportions of adult blood levels that reveal high cholesterol, high triglycerides, and abnormal glucose scores.

The American Medical Association has announced that a diet lower in fats can and does reverse the damage done by years of a high-fat, high-cholesterol diet. An exciting study of a woman, age fifty-four, who suffered from hyperlipidemic dementia demonstrated such a reversal. In short, she suffered from a deterioration of her mental state caused by excessive fats in her system. When her fats were reduced with diet and a drug (fenofibrate), her dementia improved dramatically.

A second study was conducted on 146 patients with multiple sclerosis. For an average of 17.1 years they were placed on a low-fat diet. The result was that the course of their disease was less rapidly progressive than in untreated cases. There was a significant reduction in death rate, in the frequency and severity of the aggravation of their condition, and in the rate at which patients became unable to walk or work. When treated early in their disease, a high percentage of these patients remained unchanged for up to twenty years. It was also observed that the benefits were greater for those who consumed more fluid oils than solid fats than in those who consumed solid fat over fluid oils.

Case History

The experience of Dale Harris is a good example of how excessive fat in the diet can wreck a body and of how a vigorous change in diet and lifestyle can improve what would seem to be a hopeless case. For most of his life, Dale had eaten "high on the hog"; steaks, hamburgers, eggs, bacon, and cheese were some of his favorite foods.

They took their toll. These foods caused atherosclerosis and the plugged arteries caused misery. Before he had checked into the Whitaker Wellness Institute for a lifestyle change, he had already had a bypass operation on his heart arteries and had had the large artery carrying blood to his legs replaced with a plastic graft.

Even after this, he still did not change his diet, and these surgeries did not end his problems. He developed anginal pain again in his heart and the plastic graft to his legs began to fill up with cholesterol deposits. He could only walk a few yards before pain in his legs would force him to stop. At this point, the surgeons had run out of options and Dale was almost out of time.

He was put on the diet in this book and started on a walking program. He was also put on 500 milligrams of niacin each meal. This amount of niacin will initially cause flushing of the skin, experienced as redness and tingling, mostly on the face and upper body. This flush is caused by the release of histamine induced by niacin. After continued therapy with niacin, the flush diminishes. In addition, a single aspirin taken a half hour before niacin will eliminate most of this reaction.

When Dale entered the Institute his blood cholesterol level was 324 milligrams per cubic centimeter, triglycerides 413, HDL cholesterol 43, and blood pressure 130/78. He could hardly walk, but he improved rapidly. In two weeks his cholesterol dropped to 130, triglycerides to 123, HDL cholesterol to 37, and blood pressure to 108/66.

He took this program home with him and in two years he was fully active, walking two-and-one-half miles per day with persistently lowered blood-fat levels. He used the total program to regain his health!

THE EFFECT OF EXCESS SUGAR

Sugar refers to the simple carbohydrates, such as white sugar, brown sugar, raw sugar, and even honey. These carbohydrates are absorbed immediately into the bloodstream. As discussed previously, excess carbohydrates can be converted into triglycerides to congest the bloodstream. Simple carbohydrates are converted at once, while complex carbohydrates (from grain, vegetables, and fruit) require 27 percent of the calorie content to make this conversion. In contrast to sugar, complex carbohydrates are less concentrated since they are combined with fiber, vitamins, and minerals, and are more appropriately proportioned to your body's needs and ability to handle them properly. Complex carbohydrates do not contribute as much to blood-sugar levels or body fat as simple sugars do.

When simple carbohydrates like sugar are ingested, not only do they convert to fat (both in the blood and in body fat), but researchers have found that circulating cholesterol increases—specifically the form linked with atherosclerosis. The mechanism for this increase in cholesterol brought on by sugar is not known specifically, but is probably caused by increased production of cholesterol by the liver.

Carbohydrates and the Diabetic

For most of this century, the diabetic patient has been advised to avoid carbohydrates in the diet. The reasoning is clear. Since carbohydrates are broken down into glucose before entering the bloodstream, and since the single most obvious abnormality of the diabetic condition is an elevated blood-glucose level, commonsense would dictate that carbohydrates should be avoided. In the 1920s and 1930s, the Woodyatt diet, containing 78 percent fat, 7 percent protein, and only 14 percent carbohydrate calories, was widely utilized—disastrous for those put on it. Over the years, it was found that diabetics regularly died of many complications from such a high-fat, high-cholesterol diet. Heart disease is at least twice as common in diabetics as in the general population, and 75 percent to 85 percent of all diabetics in the United States still die of atherosclerotic lesions.

Fortunately, the truth is now known, and most diabetics are instructed to consume 55 to 60 percent of their total calories in complex carbohydrates, 12 to 20 percent in protein, and no more than 35 percent in fat. However, the optimal diet composition for the diabetic would be the 68 percent complex carbohydrates, 12 percent protein, and 20 percent fat recommended in this book.

Complex carbohydrates, rather than a cause of diabetes, work to eliminate or prevent the condition from occurring. Carbohydrates in the diet make the body more sensitive to the insulin that is produced in the pancreas. This takes the stress off the pancreas, as the body handles the complex carbohydrates with less insulin than would be necessary if they were restricted in the diet. The diabetic should choose carbohydrate foods like breads, cereals, vegetables, potatoes, and fruits, which all contain a large amount of dietary fiber.

THE EFFECT OF EXCESS SALT

When we discuss excess salt (sodium chloride) in the diet, we also include such additives as monosodium glutamate, baking soda (sodium bicarbonate), and all other ingredients with "sodium" as part of their name.

When there is excess sodium in the diet, more fluid in the blood is necessary to dilute the extra sodium. This causes edema, as the fluid accumulates in the body tissues. This extra fluid can increase your blood volume and the water in and around your cells, causing your feet to swell, rings to tighten, and your eyelids to become puffy.

Obviously, if you consume salt on an occasional basis (such as salty popcorn at the movies), your body could restore the proper equilibrium and there would be no overt signs of excess sodium. However, as is typical in America, we consume excess salt on a daily basis, even from meal to meal. The body cannot restore the balance with such a continuous onslaught.

If you suffer from edema, your doctor might prescribe a diuretic. This is a dangerous way to handle a dietary problem, as the side effects of diuretics are far more dangerous than temporary edema fluid. In addition, the diuretic treats only the symptoms of the problem and does not address the real problem—too much salt!

Hypertension is attributed to imbalances in the diet of sodium, as well as of potassium and calcium. It is also linked to other factors, both external and internal—heredity, race, obesity, smoking, drugs like caffeine or decongestants, stress/type-A personality, alcohol abuse, and a sedentary lifestyle. All have been proven to a degree. We are all individuals who respond to internal and external influences in varying ways. However, the excess sodium and inadequate potassium intake of the American diet is the primary cause of high blood pressure for most people, and this problem is not of small dimensions.

High blood pressure affects an estimated 23 million Americans. If your blood pressure reading is above 140 over 90 while you are at rest, you have high blood pressure. Hypertension can lead to blindness, kidney failure, heart attacks, or stroke. The frightening thing about high blood pressure is that there usually are no symptoms. It is the kind of disease that can sneak up and do damage with a massive stroke. There is only one way to find out about your blood pressure, and that is to have it taken regularly. If it is above 140 over 90, think "potassium foods." Talk to your doctor about changing your diet before you resort to medication.

HOW TO STOP EXCESSES IN THE DIET

If you are one of those people who never gave a thought to the effect of your food choices, perhaps by now you have become aware of the power you have over your ultimate destiny. The menus and recipes in this book have been designed to help you eat deliciously and defensively. All recipes have a nutritional breakdown, so you can really understand what you are eating. Put the salt shaker, sugar bowl, and butter dish away. That step alone will help you to normalize your blood profile.

6

A Doctor's Program for Successful Weight Control

There's no single factor that can affect your blood chemistry as much as obesity. It shows up in blood tests as high cholesterol levels, high triglyceride levels, and often causes high glucose levels, reflecting the excessive fat and sugar consumption of most obese people.

However, Dr. Jean Mayer, in a five-part newspaper series on obesity, accurately points out that mild obesity by itself, with no other complications, is not a major risk factor in heart disease. So, for some, mild obesity may be more a cosmetic problem than a health problem. Never assume that obesity is the major indicator of impending heart attack. Many thin men with elevated blood-cholesterol levels have gone to the grave prematurely from heart attacks.

What both the thin person and the obese person need to do is eat the *right* foods. Generally speaking, the foods that cause a heavy person's obesity are the same foods that contribute to such problems as elevated triglycerides, elevated cholesterol, and elevated blood glucose. These, of course, lead to atherosclerosis, coronary heart disease, and diabetes. In fact, the wrong foods contribute to all degenerative diseases.

But why is obesity such a problem in this country? Thousands of books on obesity have come and gone, yet according to Metropolitan Life's tables of optimum weight, 76 percent of men and 62 percent of women in the United States are too fat.

In fact, the problem of obesity is swelling. According to statistics compiled by the National Center for Health Statistics, the average American adult in 1980 was 6 pounds heavier than the average adult was in 1960. Why?

The answer is right under our nose, and it is not the obvious answer. We do not eat too much food, we just eat the *wrong kind* of food.

Did you ever wonder why the Japanese, who are as affluent as we are, have almost no obesity problem? Do they perpetually diet? No. Do they obsessively exercise? No, you hardly see a jogger in Japan. Are they genetically protected? No. When they come to this country, they soon struggle with obesity just like the rest of us.

Does that mean that the Japanese, on the trip over, lose their dietary discipline, and then gain weight? Not likely. They eat as much food as they want in Japan, just as they do here. The difference, however, lies in the type of calories they eat, not the amount. In Japan, they eat more carbohydrate calories but less fat calories than Americans:

PERCENTAGE OF CALORIES

	Carbohydrate	Fat	Protein
Japanese	70	15	15
Americans	43	40	17

This compositional shift seems to be the reason for the lack of obesity in Japanese society and is probably the solution to the obesity problem in this country for several reasons.

EAT CARBOHYDRATES, LOSE WEIGHT

When you eat more carbohydratess, you eat fewer calories naturally, without dieting, and lose weight.

In a recent study from the Division of Nutritional Sciences at Cornell University in Ithaca, New York, Lauren Lissner, Ph.D., and colleagues found that replacing fat calories with carbohydrate calories caused a natural reduction in caloric intake. A group of twenty-four women were allowed to eat as much food as they wanted over two-week periods in which the percentage of fat calories was controlled. During the first two weeks, fat contributed 15 to 20 percent of the total calories, the second week 30 to 35 percent, and the fourth week 45 to 50 percent of the calories. The food was made equally palatable and satisfying and no calorie restrictions were imposed.

When the volunteers were eating the 15-to-20-percent fat-calorie regimen, their caloric intake was found to be 2,125 calories. On the 30-to-35-percent fat-calorie regimen the caloric intake rose to 2,375 calories, and on the high-fat regimen, 40 to 50 percent caloric fat, the women were consuming 2,750 calories per day.

Weight changes that occurred during each two-week regimen were significantly different. On the low-fat regimen, the women lost an average of .4 kilograms (about nine-tenths of a pound), on the medium-fat intake weight loss was .03 kilograms (very little, under one-tenth of a pound), and on the high-fat intake there was a weight *gain* of .32 kilograms (seven-tenths of a pound).

Without calorie restrictions there was significant weight loss accomplished

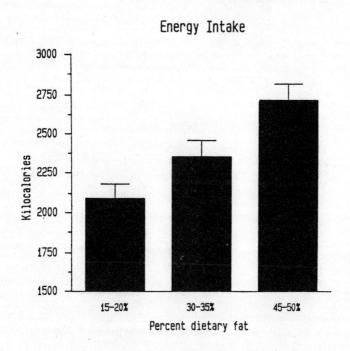

Average daily energy intake over 14 days. Reprinted with permission of the *American Journal of Clinical Nutrition*, vol. 46: p. 886, 1987.

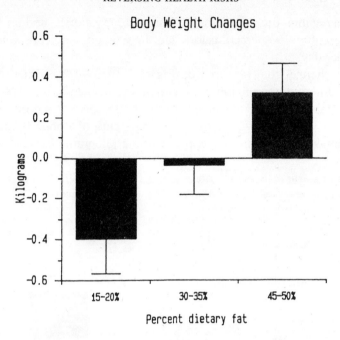

Average change in body over the 14-day experiment. Reprinted with permission of the *American Journal of Clinical Nutrition*, vol. 46: p.886, 1987.

simply by reducing the amount of fat consumed and replacing that fat with carbohydrates.

The researchers concluded:

> Altering the type of food consumed (significant reduction in fat calories) can induce spontaneous weight loss in both obese and non-obese individuals. Reduction of habitual fat intake appears to be a promising approach because it imposes no limitations on the quantity of foods consumed, but rather, emphasizes the selection of low fat foods. It seems likely that such *qualitative* changes may be more

readily incorporated into an individual's lifestyle. (*American Journal of Clinical Nutrition*, Vol. 46:886–92, 1987.)

CARBOHYDRATES ARE NOT FATTENING

Complex carbohydrates (fresh fruits, vegetables, whole grains, breads, beans, and potatoes) must not be blamed for obesity. Simple carbohydrates (white sugar, honey, and syrups) and refined carbohydrates (white flour and its products) have given carbohydrates a bad reputation.

People who avoid complex-carbohydrate foods because they are "starchy" are making a big mistake. Compared to fats, carbohydrates contain only 4 calories per gram, while a gram of fat contains 9. Since fat is more calorically concentrated than carbohydrates, a little overeating of fatty foods represents more than double the calories of protein and carbohydrates. In addition, complex carbohydrates contain fiber, which fills the intestinal tract and acts as a natural barrier to overeating. For example, how many baked potatoes (without butter or sour cream) could you eat? How many apples? If you were to eat extra potatoes, without all the fatty toppings, you would lose weight very rapidly and not feel hungry.

In addition, dietary fat is easily stored, requiring only 3 percent of its calories to transport the fat into storage cells. Carbohydrates must be converted to fat before storage, and the whole process takes 27 percent of the calories present, an inefficient exercise.

Studies have shown that carbohydrates, even when ingested to excess, only rarely stimulate obesity. Only 1 to 3 percent of the carbohydrate calories ingested wind up as stored fat, even if you overeat.

Elliott Danforth, Jr., M.D., from the College of Medicine at the University of Vermont in Burlington, in an excellent summary article that pinpointed the fat in our diet as the cause of obesity, stated:

When taken in excess, fat is more fattening than carbohydrate. Therefore, the higher carbohydrate content of a diet irrespective of its caloric content, the smaller consequences of disrupting energy balance and the less efficient the gain in weight. Therefore, if one is destined to overeat and desires to suffer the least obesity, overindulgence in carbohydrate rather than fat should be recommended. This statement is obviously ridiculous, but in view of these considerations and the tendency toward overnutrition in most affluent societies, main attention should be toward reducing both caloric and fat intake. (*The American Journal of Clinical Nutrition*, V. 41: 1132–1145, 1985.)

FIBER PREVENTS OBESITY

Studies of different cultures throughout the world have consistently demonstrated that those who eat more dietary fiber have less obesity. Natural complex carbohydrates, in fact, are the only source of dietary fiber. Meats, eggs, cheese, milk, and oils have none. Fiber fills the digestive tract, and acting somewhat like a broom, sweeps through—eliminating constipation and preventing diseases like colon cancer. Fiber can literally absorb undesirable toxins from the bowel and thoroughly eliminate them with no harm done.

The nutrients in fibrous carbohydrate foods are more slowly absorbed, allowing the body time to deal with them. Fiber gives you a feeling of fullness. You eat less. Consider for example that there is approximately the same amount of sugar in twelve apples as is in one candy bar. Yet, how many apples can you eat? This vividly illustrates how easily we can overeat simple and refined carbohydrates that are mixed with fat (as in the candy bar, which is often 50 percent fat calories) and how nearly impossible it would be to overeat the complex carbohydrates in apples.

What you eat is far more important than how much. This can be qualified by explaining at the outset that when you eat the right foods, it is difficult to overeat. Consider again the example of the candy bar and the apples. The answer of course, is that one or two apples will just about do it. But two or three candy bars go down quite easily, and there is still room for pizza. This is why *what* you eat is more important than *how much* when you are concerned about obesity.

Consumed fat enters the bloodstream and is cleared from the blood by the enzyme lipoprotein lipase. The net effect of this enzyme at the cellular level on fat circulating in the blood is the storage of fat. For some, once the fat is stored in the fat cells, it becomes exceedingly difficult to get it out. Therefore, fat restriction, not calorie restriction, is the first order of business for obesity control.

LOW-CALORIE DIETS MAKE THE PROBLEM WORSE

For most people rigid low-calorie dieting as a means of weight control is like gunning your engine when your back wheels are stuck in mud. All the effort and anxiety only make the problem worse.

The commonsense edict—that you must reduce your calories to reduce your weight—no longer fits with our understanding of how the body handles carbohydrates, fats, and low-calorie diets. What does occur from prolonged or cyclic low-calorie dieting is the creation of more severe obesity.

Kelly Brownell at the University of Pennsylvania chronicled the progress of experimental rats as they gained, lost, and regained weight. After first gaining some weight, a very low-calorie diet was instituted, and it took the rats twenty-one days to lose the excess. When food was returned to their cages it took forty-six days to regain the lost weight. When the cycle was repeated, it took forty-six days, more than twice as long to relose the same weight (remember these rats couldn't "cheat"), but only fourteen days to gain it back.

"It's as though dieting teaches the body a lesson about obesity," Brownell explained to *Nutrition Action* (March, 1987). An organism that is repeatedly deprived of fat increases its chances of survival if it learns to store food more efficiently when it is available. When food is once again scarce, the body shuts down its "calorie-burning furnace."

Low-calorie dieting is like a famine to the body. The body learns to adapt to periods of scarcity by efficiently conserving calories, thus holding on to weight. The basal metabolic rate of the body drops dramatically when there is a significant reduction in calorie intake. When calories are plentiful again, the body stores the excess much more efficiently, and usually individuals gain more weight than they lost.

Case History

In the Newport Beach, California, area, a prominent businessman was eating several meals a week in a popular Italian restaurant. He was about thirty pounds overweight. He met with the chef, who agreed to prepare for him a pasta dish with a simple sauce of tomatoes, basil, oregano, and other vegetables and herbs. No oils or other fats were used. The pasta meal was always pleasant, and he enjoyed it two times a day for about two months. He lost twenty-five pounds and *never felt deprived.*

EXERCISE AND OBESITY

Other than sumo wrestlers (who force-feed themselves for desired effect), professional bowlers, and professional golfers, the overwhelming majority of professional athletes are quite lean. How often do you see a professional tennis match between men with pot bellies? Can you imagine a competitive figure skater with a fat stomach? Exercise is a powerful tool for weight control because it "stokes the furnace." Oftentimes, simply instituting regular exercise will cause substantial weight loss without a diet change.

When you are walking briskly or riding a bicycle, you are burning close to 8 calories per minute above the caloric expenditure of your body at rest. Therefore, thirty minutes of walking per day will burn an additional 240 calories which, over a thirty-day period, would equal 7,200 calories. If all of these additional calories were derived from stored body fat, this amount of activity would burn up about 800 grams, about 1.6 pounds.

But as most exercise physiologists will confirm, this level of activity stimulates far more weight loss than the expected weight loss generated by the exercise itself. This is because when you exercise, you increase the basal metabolic rate for several hours after the activity.

WEIGHT LOSS PRINCIPLES: YOUR KEY TO COMPLETE CONTROL OF YOUR WEIGHT

- Don't use your discipline to count calories. Discipline is a powerful force, and if you are going to use it, use it where it will do the most good. Eat until you are satisfied; just do not "overeat."
- Eliminate excess fat from your diet. Follow the recipes in the back of this book, which are calculated to give you about 1,600 calories a day with only 20 percent of those calories coming from fat.
- When you are hungry, snack on fresh fruit, preferably the succulent fruits like apples or pears. Eat as many apples as you want (just how many could you eat?).
- Start taking vitamin and mineral supplements to insure that your metabolic systems are supplied with all the nutrients for optimal function.
- Start an exercise program and use some of that precious discipline to keep it going.

Sample:

Week One: Walk five minutes from your house and back per day at a moderate pace.

Week Two: Increase this to ten minutes (twenty minutes round trip) at the same moderate pace.

Week Three: Increase this to fifteen minutes (thirty minutes round trip) at the same pace.

Week Four: Increase the pace so that you cover about 10 percent more ground.

Week Five: Walk at a pace that will cause your pulse to elevate to about 70 percent of your maximum calculated pulse rate. (See chapter 8. The maximum calculated pulse rate is derived by subtracting your age from 220.)

By this time you should be feeling pretty well, and it is best to have one or two days of rest during the week. Congratulations.

There you have it—the keys to successful weight control.

HOW WEIGHT LOSS AFFECTS THE BLOOD LEVEL

Weight loss and successful weight control alter the blood profile in the most healthy way. Almost every important aspect of the blood test is improved by a successful weight-loss and weight-control program.

First, the fasting blood-sugar level invariably falls. In fact, successful weight loss is so helpful in bringing down the blood-sugar level that it is the only method of treatment for certain forms of diabetes. This form of diabetes, non-insulin-dependent diabetes, invariably improves with successful weight loss. Millions of men and women who are currently taking oral medications such as Micronase, Diabinese, and even insulin could become drug-free with normal blood-sugar levels if they follow the above program for successful weight loss.

The next most important area affected in a beneficial way by weight loss is in blood-fat measurements. Weight loss invariably will cause a drop in the blood-triglyceride level, the measurement of neutral fat. Along with the drop in neutral fat will be very significant drops in the total cholesterol and LDL cholesterol, the most dependable predictors of heart disease. In addition, weight loss tends to elevate HDL cholesterol, further decreasing the risk of heart disease.

Weight loss affects the blood–uric acid level as well. As we have discussed, uric-acid elevation can stimulate arthritis and is a little-appreciated risk factor for heart disease. Successful weight loss will cause a drop in the uric-acid level, decreasing the risk of arthritis and heart disease at the same time.

However, rapid weight loss will cause a transient increase in the uric-acid level and should be avoided. The principles for weight loss above avoid this tendency toward rapid weight reduction, insuring moderate yet continuous weight loss until optimal weight is achieved. As a result, the chances for transient elevation of the uric-acid level are diminished.

In addition, successful weight loss will substantially lower the blood pressure. Like men and women who suffer from non-insulin-dependent diabetes, most of those who are obese and have high blood pressure can likewise become drug-free if the weight-loss principles are used successfully. This would not only save millions of dollars currently spent for high-blood-pressure medications, but would also eliminate the side effects of those drugs in the many obese people who currently take them to control their blood pressure.

Successful weight loss and weight control also improve the intracellular concentrations of magnesium and potassium. The concentration of these minerals tends to increase within the cell after successful weight loss, and, as mentioned previously, this is a very healthy change.

Not only do positive changes occur in objective tests of health, but studies have shown that, psychologically, successful weight control is a major boost to self-confidence and an overall sense of well-being. As you begin to feel more comfortable with your body, you will likely begin to take a greater interest in sex and enjoy it more.

The new principles of concentrating on fat restriction and exercise instead of rigid calorie control certainly make it possible for more people to achieve and maintain optimal weight than in the past.

Successful Weight Control: The Payoff

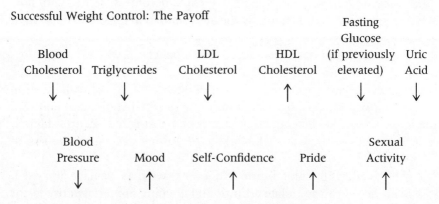

Blood Cholesterol	Triglycerides	LDL Cholesterol	HDL Cholesterol	Fasting Glucose (if previously elevated)	Uric Acid
↓	↓	↓	↑	↓	↓

Blood Pressure	Mood	Self-Confidence	Pride	Sexual Activity
↓	↑	↑	↑	↑

——— 7 ———

Vitamins and Trace Mineral Levels: A Secret of Healthy Blood Chemistry

In the name of self-preservation, it's important to know as much as possible about the vitamin and mineral content of your food supply. While research is being conducted all over the world to determine how nutrients can give you a protective benefit, there is a great deal already known about the effect of vitamins and minerals upon the body. Yet questions are being asked by consumers faster than science seems to come up with the answers. In promoting wellness a new emphasis on prevention and a greater interest in the problems that can occur when there are insufficient vitamins or an imbalance of minerals are having an impact on the medical community. These nutrients or lack of them can literally affect your health potential.

VITAMINS AND MINERALS AS COFACTORS FOR ENZYMES

Vitamins and minerals are essential nutrients because they are needed as cofactors for enzymes, which speed up the digestion of food. A cofactor can be likened to a key, and the enzyme can represent the lock; without the key in the lock the function of the enzyme cannot take place. Each enzyme has a highly specific job to do, and each has a need for specific keys (in this case, certain vitamins and minerals) to enable the enzyme to give the action and reaction that is needed. If you've got the nutrient, the enzyme performs. If the nutrient isn't available, the function of the enzyme doesn't occur. If all receptor sites for the required vitamin or mineral on the enzymes are filled, the enzymes are "saturated" and can perform their tasks. Any excess vitamins and minerals that are ingested will have to be stored in the liver or eliminated by the body. To add to the guesswork of vitamin intake, each person has unique requirements, some using more energy and needing to replace it with enzymatic action more often than others.

Enzymes are proteins that are part of your inherited genes and are present in every cell. When they function as expected, you can be in a state of optimal health. When there is a deprivation of the vitamins and minerals needed by enzymes to complete a specific metabolic reaction, a state of subnormal health patterns begin to appear. Such subnutrition may never cause you to reach a point of obvious clinical deterioration, but it can sap your health away at an undetected sublevel for years and years.

Most mineral elements contribute to two general body functions of building and regulating—building skeletal and soft tissues, or regulating such systems as heartbeat, blood clotting, internal pressure of body fluids, and transport of oxygen from the lungs to the tissues (which you will remember is done by the red blood cells).

Excess vitamins are either stored (fat-soluble) or voided (water-soluble), but excess minerals may upset the balance and function of other minerals in the body, contributing to such health problems as anemia, bone demineralization and breakage, neurological dysfunction, and fetal abnormalities. People who take mineral supplements should not use them in amounts greatly in excess of what the body requires.

BLOOD TESTS CAN REVEAL VITAMIN AND MINERAL LEVELS

Your blood profile at times can reveal an imbalance of certain essential nutrients that can affect your well-being. A magnesium deficiency indicated by low plasma levels, for example, is characteristic of heart disease, diabetes, high blood pressure, and heart arrhythmia, but, unfortunately, is frequently overlooked.

Low blood-selenium levels have been associated with an increased incidence of cardiovascular disease. Studies with rats show that selenium may also play a role in cancer prevention.

A zinc deficiency may result in dermatitis, diarrhea, increased susceptibility to infections, stunting of growth, and difficult childbirths. In a study of Scandinavian women at mid-pregnancy, women who had abnormal labor also showed lower levels of plasma zinc.

Iron deficiency can lead to anemia, a condition of low red-blood-cell count.

96

Since red blood cells carry oxygen to every cell in the body, a low count means an inadequate supply of oxygen. This can leave many cells gasping for oxygen and functioning at subnormal levels.

A specific vitamin or mineral deficiency can be determined in two ways. First, there are blood tests that can be used to screen for deficiency of either vitamins or minerals. These tests are not regularly used but are available. Very few laboratories do these tests, and they tend to be expensive.

A second method is to analyze vitamin deficiency by measuring enzyme function. Since many enzymes have vitamin coenzymes, a prolonged vitamin deficiency will reduce, if not inactivate, the enzyme function. This is particularly true with deficiencies of the B-complex family of water-soluble vitamins, since various members of the B family take part in coenzyme activity, enabling an enzyme to do its specific metabolic task.

However, a battery of tests to determine specific vitamin or mineral deficiency is not necessary before starting a supplement program. Vitamin and mineral supplements act as nutritional insurance against deficiency, and every patient at the Whitaker Wellness Institute is given a supplement regimen. The goal of supplementation is to saturate the enzyme system with coenzymes to insure optimal function. Supplementation also takes care of any genetic differences, insuring adequate nutrients across a wide range of intakes.

GOVERNMENT RDAS FOR VITAMINS AND MINERALS

Standards set by the Food and Nutrition Board of the National Academy of Sciences are the Recommended Dietary Allowances (RDA) of essential nutrients. The RDAs are by definition:

> "The levels of intake of essential nutrients considered, in the judgement of the committee on Dietary Allowances of the Food and Nutrition Board on the basis of available scientific knowledge, to be adequate to meet the known nutrional needs of practically all healthy persons."

The RDAs are recommendations established for healthy populations, not for individuals. However, individuals vary markedly from one another. In fact, it would be almost impossible to find that mythical "average person" for whom all the RDAs would be perfect. Just as we have different hair color, body size, intelligence, and personalities, we have different requirements for micronutrients of energy levels. Also consider that there are special needs for extra nutrients that occur owing to the use of oral contraceptives, pregnancy, premature birth, inherited metabolic disorders, infections, chronic diseases, the use of medications, smoking, frequent alcohol consumption, and other lifestyle choices.

DOES YOUR DIET PROVIDE ENOUGH VITAMINS AND MINERALS?

It depends on what you are eating. If you are dieting on a daily 1,000-calorie weight-loss regimen, it is hardly possible for you to assimilate the variety of nutrients you need. This is especially true if you follow the "fad diet of the month" that tells you to eat just one kind of food all day with complete disregard for your body's need for a wide range of foods to supply a diversification of nutrients.

If you are in the habit of eating a high-fat, processed-food diet, it is entirely likely that you are not getting the wide array of vitamins needed to maintain optimal health each day. Processed food strips the nutrients out during the manufacturing process. Some vitamins may be added back artificially, but not necessarily in the proportions that they appear in the natural food, and the accompanying minerals probably won't be intact either. When you are eating a high proportion of fat and a high proportion of protein every day, there's not much room left for the complex-carbohydrate group of foods that provides most of the essential vitamins and minerals your body needs in order to thrive.

WHAT ARE THE FACTS ABOUT CURRENT NUTRITION PRACTICES?

While many people are concerned with eating a nutritious diet, a large portion of the population is not meeting minimal RDA standards. According to a USDA Nationwide Food Consumption Survey in 1977–78, about one-third of Americans are consuming low-calorie diets, eating less than 70 percent of their RDA of calories needed for energy. At this level, individuals may have difficulty meeting the RDAs for vitamins and minerals. Included in this low-calorie population are 40 percent of all women aged nineteen to fifty.

The same study showed that mean intakes of calcium, iron, magnesium, and vitamin B_6 were in the range of only 40 to 60 percent of the RDA for women, girls, and boys consuming low-calorie diets. For instance, girls aged fifteen to eighteen on low-calorie diets met the RDA only for protein, among all of the nutrients studied.

In addition, it was determined that vitamin B_6 is a problem nutrient for nearly three-fourths of American women. More than half of all individuals studied had vitamin B_6 intakes below 70 percent of the RDA.

Regarding calcium, 42 percent of all individuals studied had intakes below 70 percent of the RDA. It was concluded that calcium is a problem nutrient for more than half of American women (51 to 62 percent) over eleven years of age.

Nearly a third of all people studied had vitamin A intakes below 70 percent of the RDA.

One-fourth of all individuals studied had vitamin C intakes below 70 percent of the RDA.

Eighty-two percent of infants aged one to two years and 64–73 percent of women aged twelve to fifty had iron intakes below 70 percent of the RDA.

Overall, data from the USDA 1977–78 Nationwide Food Consumption Survey indicate that vitamins B_6, A, and C, and minerals such as calcium, iron, and magnesium may be problem nutrients for a number of sex-age groups in the United States. In addition to these nutrients recognized as potential problems for the general population, there are other nutrients that may pose problems for people who continue on low-calorie diets for long periods of time.

Keeping in mind that the RDAs are just minimal goals to prevent malnutrition, we can see that these statistics point up the great need for better nutrient intake to promote better health.

It is not within the scope of this book to discuss each of the nutrional elements that are used to supplement the diet-and-exercise program at the Whitaker Wellness Institute, but rather the rationale for the supplementation and for the concentrations that are contained in the recommendations.

As mentioned above, the recommended daily allowances do not take into account the significant variability that exists between individuals. Dr. Roger Williams, the world-renowned nutrional scientist who discovered pantothenic acid, has been advocating nutritional supplements for the last thirty-five years as a form of "nutritional insurance." When you buy fire insurance for your home, you do not wish for your home to burn down. Likewise, nutritional supplements act as insurance guarding against inadequate intake of the essential nutrients caused by either the processed foods of civilization or inborn genetic differences between individuals.

The supplement formula used at the Whitaker Wellness Institute supplies the nutrients at moderate elevations to cover the nutrient requirements of almost everyone adequately.

There is very little potential of toxicity from this nutrient formula for the following reasons. Both the water-soluble nutrients (the B-complex vitamins and vitamin C) and the fat-soluble elements (vitamin A, vitamin E, and vitamin D) are given in doses at which there have been no significant reports of toxicity. However, the concentration of this formula is such that it not only supplies adequate nutrition, but is also at a dosage level that can be therapeutic to those who are suffering with an illness and aid in regaining their health.

VITAMIN GUIDE

Vitamin A

Vitamin A is needed to protect eyesight, prevent night blindness, and maintain the skin and mucous membranes. The beta-carotene found in carrots is thought to be protective against cancer. A mild vitamin-A deficiency is associated with a rise in respiratory disease, diarrhea, and thyroid problems. Vitamin A affects absorption, digestion, healing, and the rebuilding of tissues.

Beta-carotene is the plant form of vitamin A. Carotenoids are only active if they can be converted to retinol during or subsequent to absorption through the intestinal wall. Preformed vitamin A is found in animal products such as liver, milk, and eggs, while "provitamin A" carotenoids are found in yellow and dark green leafy vegetables and in some fruits like yellow melons.

Vitamin B-Complex

Vitamin B-complex is needed to maintain the nervous system in the production of neurotransmitters, to build and repair muscles, and to produce energy.

Thiamine (B_1) is essential for the integrity of the central nervous system, muscle coordination, and the metabolism of carbohydrates and proteins. It is involved in the synthesis of nerve-regulating substances. It combines with manganese as a coenzyme. It is not stored in the body in great quantity. Depletion is caused by smoking and drinking alcoholic beverages. Alcohol interferes with the absorption of thiamine, causing an eventual deficiency in heavy drinkers.

A deficiency of thiamine can cause gastrointestinal problems, cardiac derangement, a weakened heart muscle, enlarged heart, congestive heart failure, swelling, polyneuritis, and, in extreme cases, causes beriberi.

The human body's requirement for thiamine is related to energy intake. The need increases with the increased consumption of carbohydrates. Elevated body temperature will also raise the thiamine requirement, as will pregnancy, lactation, and the use of birth control pills.

Riboflavin (B₂) functions in the release of energy to cells from carbohydrates, proteins, and fats. It is important in the maintenance of mucous membranes and for protecting against eye disorders.

Riboflavin is a coenzyme that combines with phosphoric acid. Mild deficiency can cause burning of skin and eyes, headaches, mental depression, cracking at angles of the mouth, scaly dermatitis around the nose opening, and can affect the cornea of the eye.

It is often difficult to isolate signs of riboflavin deficiency from those of other B-vitamin deficiencies because B vitamins are generally found together in the same foods. Generally, treatment for this deficiency involves supplementation with the entire B-complex rather than with riboflavin alone.

Riboflavin was identified as a growth-promoting factor in yeast extracts in 1920, then later chemically identified and synthesized in 1935.

Niacin (B₃) is needed for metabolic processes such as the conversion of food to energy, fat synthesis, protein metabolism, and tissue respiration. Niacin is also involved in mental health and mucous-membrane integrity.

A deficiency of niacin can cause gastrointestinal problems, mucous-membrane problems, mental problems, muscle weakness, and at its greatest deficiency will cause pellagra. Pellagra is a disease in which the skin forms a reddish rash which later turns dark and rough.

The body can obtain adequate niacin by converting dietary tryptophan (an amino acid found in proteins) to nicotinic acid. This conversion depends on the presence of other amino acids and vitamins B_1, B_6, and biotin in the diet.

Pyridoxine (B₆) is necessary for amino-acid metabolism in the synthesis of serotonin from tryptophan in brain chemistry, for the proper functioning of the nervous system, and to maintain sodium/potassium intracellular balance. It is also needed for the absorption of B_{12}, for production of hydrochloric acid, antibodies, and red blood cells.

There is good evidence that vitamin-B_6 deficiency may be a problem for alcoholics because alcohol interferes with the body's utilization of vitamin B_6. There is also some evidence that users of birth-control pills may have an increased need for pyridoxine, as 15 to 20 percent of oral-contraceptive users show direct biochemical evidence of vitamin-B_6 deficiency.

Vitamin B_6 has been found to relieve symptoms of bronchial asthma, although the findings are preliminary. However, B_6 is not a cure for asthma.

Some signs of severe vitamin-B_6 deficiency in adults may be depression, confusion, and abnormal brain waves followed by convulsions. Other symptoms include inflammation of the mucous membranes in the mouth, inflammation of the tongue, fissures and scaling of the lips and corners of the mouth, and patches of itchy, scaling skin.

Deficiency of pyridoxine can cause infants to convulse or may cause weight loss, abdominal distress, vomiting, and hyperirritability.

Vitamin B_{12} (cobalamin) is needed for red blood cells, for the healthy functioning of all cells, for the production of hydrochloric acid, and for protection of the myelin sheath of the spine. It is also necessary in the synthesis of DNA.

While dietary deficiency of vitamin B_{12} is rare, except in some elderly patients and in some strict vegetarians, it may be caused by a problem with absorption. Deficiency of vitamin B_{12} causes megaloblastosis (refusal of a cell to divide). It can cause anemia, growth disorder, constipation, demyelination of the spinal cord, and paralysis.

Folic Acid (folacin) is needed for DNA and growth. A folate deficiency can cause irritability, hostility, paranoid behavior, and gastrointestinal diseases.

Severe folacin deficiency leads to impaired cell division and altered protein synthesis. Megaloblastic anemia, a disease marked by the presence of abnormal red blood cells in the bone marrow, and macrocytic anemia, a disease marked by oversized red blood cells, are also signs of severe deficiency. Macrocytic anemia may also reveal a decrease in the number of white blood cells, a condition called leukopenia.

Pantothenic Acid is a peptidelike compound that is essential in the metabolism of fats and proteins and for the release of energy from carbohydrates. It is also necessary for the formation of hormones and other vital compounds that regulate the nervous system.

Although dietary deficiency of pantothenic acid is still under experimentation, it is thought that such deficiency can result in headache, fatigue, impaired motor coordination, prickling or tingling of the skin, muscle cramps, and gastrointestinal disturbances.

Biotin is necessary in the metabolism of carbohydrates, fats, and proteins. Besides being readily available in all plant and animal foods, biotin is synthesized by intestinal bacteria. For this reason, it is rare to have a dietary deficiency in biotin, except in infants. When dietary deficiency is experimentally induced, the results are characterized by mild skin disorders, some anemia, depression, insomnia, and muscle pain.

Vitamin C

Vitamin C (ascorbic acid) has an antiviral effect, an antihistamine effect, and is also thought to have an anticancer effect. It is believed to protect the immune system, to have influence on the substances that hold cells together, and to help regulate intercellular reactions. It is essential for the intestinal absorption of iron, the formation of dentin, wound healing, blood clotting, and the production of neurotransmitters. It is important in the maintenance of health of bones, teeth, blood vessels, the formation of collagen, and is an antioxidant. It may also play a role in the proper functioning of white blood cells.

Vitamin C is greatly depleted by smoking, alcoholic beverages, and stress. A severe deficiency causes scurvy, a potentially fatal disease.

Ascorbic acid is sensitive to heat, air, and water, and thus may be destroyed during overcooking or by cooking in too much water.

Vitamin D

Vitamin D is necessary in bone growth, and in the repair and maintenance of bones. It is especially necessary for the absorption of calcium, and promotes the absorption of phosphates and phosphorus.

Vitamin-D deficiency in children causes rickets, a disease that twists and bends bones. In adults, vitamin-D deficiency causes bones to lose their density. Elderly people suffer from this condition, and it is believed that inadequate vitamin D may play an important role in the development of osteoporosis.

Vitamin E

Vitamin E is an antioxidant, helping to prevent the ravages of aging. Vitamin E protects fat-containing membranes found in the nerves, muscles, and cardiovascular system. It helps to prolong the life of red blood cells and is also involved with the body's utilization of vitamin A.

Some evidence indicates that vitamin E may have a therapeutic role in fibrocystic disease of the breast, progressive neuromuscular disease in children, heart disease, and premenstrual syndrome (PMS). In environmental studies with animals, vitamin E has also been shown to help protect against pollutants and cigarette smoke.

Although vitamin E is considered to be helpful for cardiac health, supplementation should be raised gradually, as it can elevate blood pressure when taken suddenly in very high doses.

Dietary deficiency of vitamin E is rare, and no clinical symptoms of vitamin E deficiency have been noted. Laboratory studies have revealed biochemical changes possibly caused by vitamin-E deficiency that include shortened red-cell survival time, muscle loss, and an increased production of age pigment in certain tissues. It has been associated with, though not considered a cause of, several types of genetic blood diseases, including sickle-cell disease.

There are at least eight naturally occurring forms of vitamin E called tocopherols. Of these, alpha-tocopherol is the most common form and also has the highest biological activity.

VITAMIN AND MINERAL TOXICITY

Excess water-soluble vitamins are washed out of the body in the urine. Excess fat-soluble vitamins are stored in the body and can build up to toxic levels. The object is to get enough vitamins through food and supplementation to permit the body to thrive without taking an excess amount.

The water-soluble vitamins are the Bs and C. When taken in food and supplemented with reasonable amounts, there should be no side effects. However, there have been some instances of side effects when water-soluble B vitamins were taken in extremely high supplemental doses, making it wise to stay within recommended ranges unless a physician is prescribing a therapeutic dosage.

Fat-soluble vitamins are A, D, E, and K. Excessive levels of the fat-soluble vitamins can accumulate in body tissues and organs. With vitamins A and D, this can cause a potential for toxicity. Vitamin A in the diet is obtained from both retinol or preformed vitamin A in animal foods, and from provitamin-A carotenoids, mostly beta-carotene, in plant foods. Adverse effects have been reported from the retinols, not the carotenes. Vitamin-A toxicity from retinol can be either acute or chronic. Acute toxicity can result from very high doses over a few days, whereas chronic toxicity can result from continued use of moderately high doses for months or years. Either type of toxicity can be averted by withdrawal of excess vitamin A, taking from one to several months to recover.

Vitamin D has greater potential for toxicity than any other vitamin. High doses over a long period can lead to irreversible calcification of soft tissues such as kidneys, blood vessels, heart, lungs, and tissues around the joints. Besides this, it is possible to suffer from loss of appetite, weakness, and constipation from excess intake of vitamin D.

Vitamin E in extremely high levels can interfere with anticoagulant therapy, so patients taking vitamin E on their own and also taking medication such as Coumadin should be sure to discuss dosages with their physician. In addition, there might be gastrointestinal disturbances from vitamin E toxicity, and it is thought that high dosages can increase blood pressure in some people.

MACROMINERALS AND MICROMINERALS

Macrominerals are those needed in large amounts in the diet. They are present in large amounts in the body and are required at more than 100 milligrams each per day. The macrominerals are calcium, phosphorus, sodium, chloride, potassium, magnesium, and sulfur.

Microminerals, or trace minerals, are needed in small amounts. They are chromium, iron, manganese, copper, iodine, zinc, cobalt, fluorine, selenium, and possibly others.

Macrominerals

Calcium has the largest concentration in the body of any mineral. Almost all of the two or three pounds present in the body is in the bones and teeth. Calcium helps to regulate some body processes, such as the normal behavior of the nervous system, muscle tone, and blood clotting. In fact, calcium is essential for healthy blood and helps to regulate the heartbeat.

While elderly women are considered to be at greatest risk for osteoporosis (loss of bone mass), everyone needs calcium throughout life, although growing children and pregnant and lactating women have the highest needs. When not enough calcium is available in the diet, it is leached from the bones. If calcium is withdrawn from the bones for a prolonged period, it will result in weakened, porous bones. This condition in turn will result in a fragile bone structure that can fracture at the slightest fall or from any abrupt movement. Weight-bearing exercise, such as walking, jogging, and bicycling, will help to strengthen bones. While osteoporosis is usually seen in older patients, bone-mass loss may begin as early as age twenty when there is a calcium deficiency present.

The best sources of calcium are milk and milk products. To avoid excess fat intake, use skim milk and low-fat cheese. Other good sources of calcium are grean leafy vegetables, canned sardines, and salmon.

Magnesium is found in all body tissues, but mostly in the bones. It is necessary for enzyme conversions in the body. Generally, if you eat a wide variety of foods, you get enough magnesium; however, alcoholism and disease conditions may cause a deficiency.

People who are under a great deal of stress are also at risk of depleting magnesium. A magnesium deficiency that shows up in low plasma levels can result in such symptoms as convulsions and cardiac arrhythmia.

Magnesium is found in seafood, whole grains, dark-green vegetables, molasses, and nuts.

Phosphorus is present with calcium in the bones and teeth, and is necessary for every tissue in the body. It is widely available in a balanced diet.

Potassium is mainly in the fluid inside the body cells, where it helps to regulate fluid balance and volume. A deficiency can occur from prolonged bouts of diarrhea or from taking diuretics.

Sodium and *chloride* are combined in table salt as sodium chloride but have separate functions in the body. Sodium is found in fluids outside the body cells, acting with potassium inside the cells to maintain body-fluid balance. Sodium is also found in blood plasma. High sodium intake can contribute to hypertension, kidney disease, cirrhosis of the liver, and congestive heart disease.

Chloride is part of hydrochloric acid, which is concentrated in the gastric juice and plays a major role in digestion of food in the stomach.

Sulfur is present in all body tissues and, as a component of several important amino acids, is related to protein nutrition. Sulfur is also part of thiamine and biotin. The complete function of sulfur in the body has not been established.

Microminerals

Chromium is involved with glucose utilization. A deficiency can produce a diabetes-like condition. Chromium is found in dried brewer's yeast, whole-grain cereals, and liver.

Cobalt is part of vitamin B_{12}, an essential nutrient. Because cobalt exists only in trace amounts in plants, vegetarians who do not eat any meat, eggs, or dairy products may become deficient in this trace mineral.

Copper is involved in the formation of hemoglobin from iron. It is found in organ meats, shellfish, nuts, legumes, molasses, and raisins.

Fluorine is found in water, soil, plants, and animals. Fluoride contributes to tooth formation and is effective in preventing dental caries. There is some evidence that fluoride is helpful in retaining calcium in the bones of the elderly. The acceptable level of fluoride in drinking water is only one part per million.

Iodine is needed in very small amounts, but normal functioning of the thyroid gland depends on an adequate supply. When there is a deficiency of dietary iodine, thyroid enlargement, known as goiter, occurs. Soil in inland areas often contain little iodine, but iodized salt and seafood can supply what is needed.

Iron is necessary for the transportation of oxygen to the cells. It is widely distributed in the body, particularly in the blood, liver, spleen, and bone marrow. Loss of blood can cause an iron-deficiency anemia.

Manganese is necessary for normal tendon and bone structure and is also part of some enzymes. A deficiency in humans is unknown because it is found abundantly in many foods, especially bran, coffee, tea, nuts, peas, and beans.

Selenium is thought to have a "sparing action" on vitamin E. It has been demonstrated in animals that when there is a deficiency of either vitamin E or selenium, either nutrient can provide a cure.

Zinc is an important part of the enzymes that move carbon dioxide, via red blood cells, from the tissues to the lungs where it can be exhaled. It is also thought that zinc deficiency may be related to a loss of sense of taste and may have an effect on wound healing.

OTHER NUTRIENTS THAT ARE ATTRACTING SCIENTIFIC ATTENTION

Researchers are learning new facts every day about the way the body functions. One of the more interesting new discoveries is a substance named *coenzyme Q-10*. Coenzyme Q-10 (CoQ-10) is also known as ubiquinone. It is an important vitamin-like nutrient that resembles vitamin E and vitamin K in chemical structure. CoQ-10 is involved in the production of energy in the mitochondria located in every cell in the body, and is especially important in producing energy in heart cells.

Dr. Karl Folkers of the University of Texas is the father of CoQ-10 in the United States. He also led the research team that discovered vitamin B_{12} in 1948, and was the first to synthesize vitamin B_6. Since CoQ-10 improves energy production in heart cells, Dr. Folkers suspected in 1957 when he started his research on CoQ-10 and the heart that it would improve the heart tissue's ability to survive low-oxygen conditions, such as when arteries are clogged during a heart attack. In 1985, a study was published in the *American Journal of Cardiology* that showed CoQ-10 helped heart-attack victims and angina patients. Studies have also shown that CoQ-10 normalizes high blood pressure.

In a study of heart-attack and angina patients, researchers at Hamamatsu University in Japan led by Dr. Tadishi Kamikawa found that when patients were supplemented with CoQ-10, the number of angina attacks were cut in half, the number of nitroglycerin tablets needed were also halved, and tolerance for exercise increased by 20 percent. Other researchers have found CoQ-10 to be an effective substance for the treatment of cardiomyopathy (a disorder of the heart muscle) and congestive heart failure.

Currently, six million Japanese are using CoQ-10 as a daily supplement, usually in dosages of 10 milligrams, three times a day. Since CoQ-10 levels in the body tend to decline with age, this substance is being considered for antiaging therapy. Studies continue to show that CoQ-10 supplementation may correct some diseases associated with the aging process.

Another nutrient that is attracting attention is a unique amino acid called *L-Carnitine*. Recent research indicates that L-Carnitine plays a role in converting stored body fat into energy, controlling hypoglycemia, and that it seems to be beneficial to patients having diabetes, liver disease, and kidney disease.

L-Carnitine was originally classified as vitamin B-t, but later it was discovered that the body produces L-Carnitine from two essential amino acids (L-lysine and L-methionine) provided that vitamins B_3, B_6, and C along with iron are present in sufficient amounts.

L-Carnitine's primary role is to transport large fat molecules into the area of the cell where fats are converted into energy. It is thought that in the absence of L-Carnitine, many fats build up within the cell and the bloodstream in the form of fats and triglycerides.

An L-Carnitine deficiency causes metabolic impairment to heart tissue. Supplemental L-Carnitine has proven to be beneficial to some heart patients. According to one report in the *American Journal of Cardiology*, L-Carnitine (20 or 40 milligrams per kilogram of body weight) increased the endurance of heart patients for exercise. Other studies have shown that L-Carnitine (40 milligrams per kilogram body weight) lowers the exercise heart rate and extends the time of exercise prior to the onset of angina. When given at 100 milligrams per kilogram body weight, it reduces the number of angina attacks and nitroglycerin consumption.

MaxEPA fish oil is almost always recommended to clients at the Whitaker Wellness Institute. The health benefits of fish oil are so dramatic that it is likely that bottles of it will be as common in the American household as bottles of aspirin.

The interest in fish oil started several years ago, when it was noted that Eskimos, who consume a high-fat diet, which in other countries was known to cause heart disease, had far less heart disease than expected. The reason:

the fat from marine mammals and fish does not lead to heart attacks but seems to prevent them in two ways.

First, fish oil, even though it contains some cholesterol, actually can reduce the blood-cholesterol level as well as the blood-triglyceride level. It is more like a vegetable oil than an animal fat because it contains unsaturated bonds but differs from most vegetable oils by the location of these bonds. The unique location of the unsaturated bonds in fish oil makes it proficient in lowering blood-fat levels, particularly elevated triglycerides. In one study with ten men with dangerously high levels of both cholesterol and triglyceride, a diet high in fish oil lowered the cholesterol from 373 to 207, and the triglycerides from an average of 1,353 to 228 in only four days. (*New England Journal of Medicine*, Vol. 312:1210–6, 1985.)

Secondly, fish oil acts as a safe blood thinner by reducing the production of a substance known as thromboxane A2. This hormone, increased by animal fats in the diet, causes blood cells to stick together, thus forming dangerous clots that cause heart attacks and strokes.

In a study of thirteen men, ten capsules of fish oil per day significantly reduced production of thromboxane A2 and at the same time increased the production of another substance, prostaglandin I_3, which is a natural blood thinner. The one-two punch of blood-fat control and blood-thinning properties makes fish oil very helpful in treating and preventing heart disease.

The same effect can be obtained by eating fish two times per week. The optimal dose of fish oil depends upon the initial level of cholesterol and triglycerides, particularly the latter. A small dose could be taken by anyone indefinitely as an aid to reduce the tendency of the blood to form abnormal clots.

VITAMIN AND MINERAL CONTENT OF FOODS

Since the vitamins and minerals that are essential for us are also essential for most other forms of life, they are usually present in natural foods used by man. However, adequate amounts of vitamin B 12 and iron may not be present in a strictly vegetarian diet, so supplementation with these certainly makes sense for those who eat only vegetable foods.

In addition, numerous studies have revealed that the location of growth of the food may have a very significant effect on the nutrient content, and, as already mentioned, food storage, processing, and preparation takes its toll on the nutrients.

It is for these reasons that I would recommend vitamin and mineral supplementation as a part of your daily routine.

THE INSTITUTE'S VITAMIN AND MINERAL PROGRAM FOR OPTIMAL HEALTH

Below, is the vitamin and mineral formula that is used at the Whitaker Wellness Institute. The majority of men and women who participate in the institute programs do have symptomatic cardiovascular disease, diabetes, or high blood pressure, or a combination of these diseases. The formula below was devised to provide therapeutic levels of nutrients, but it is also ideal for prevention.

The formula is designed to saturate the enzyme systems and metabolic requirements of most men and women. Unlike the RDAs designed to prevent nutritional "deficiency," this formula is designed to provide "optimal" nutrition.

		%U.S. RDA
Beta Carotene	15,000i.u.	300
Vitamin A (Retinyl Palmitate)	5,000i.u.	100
Vitamin D_3 (Cholecalciferol)	400i.u.	100
Vitamin E (d-Alpha Tocopheryl)	400i.u.	1333
Vitamin C (Ascorbic Acid)	2,000mg	3333
Folic Acid	400mcg	100
Thiamine (Vitamin B_1)	50mg	3333
Riboflavin (Vitamin B_2)	10mg	588
Niacinamide (Vitamin B_3)	80mg	400
Niacin (Vitamin B_3)	20mg	100
Vitamin B_6 (Pyridoxine)	50mg	2500
Vitamin B_{12} (Cyanocobalamin)	40mcg	666
Biotin	300mcg	100
Calcium Pantothenate (Pantothenic Acid)	50mg	500
Choline	250mg	†
**Calcium	1,000mg	100
Iodine (Kelp)	150mcg	100
*Iron Chelate	18mg	100
***Magnesium	500mg	125
*Copper Chelate	3mg	150
*Zinc Chelate	30mg	200

****Potassium	300mg	†
*Manganese Chelate	10mg	†
*Chromium Chelate	400mcg	††
Selenium Chelate	200mcg	††
Molybdenum Chelate	150mcg	††
Silicon Chelate	20mg	††
Bioflavonoids	100mg	††
Inositol	40mg	††

Ingredients in a base of Rutin and Hesperidin.

*Each tablet contains a Mineral Protein Chelate made with specially isolated soy protein.

**Derived from Calcium Chelate, Carbonate and Gluconate

***Derived from Magnesium Chelate, Oxide and Gluconate

****Derived from Potassium Chelate and Chloride

†The need in human nutrition has been established, but no U.S. RDA has been determined.

††The need in human nutrition has not been established. U.S. RDA—United States Recommended Daily Allowance

NO YEAST, NO STARCH, NO PRESERVATIVES, NO DYES, NO SUGAR, NO SACCHARIN, NON-ALLERGENIC

A specialized formula has been devised for use at the Whitaker Wellness Institute with the intent to provide the usual doses of the major vitamins and minerals in one formula so as to avoid opening a lot of bottles. Almost all clients here use this formula while at the Institute and continue to use it at home.

For more information on this formula contact the Wellness Institute at:

4400 MacArthur Blvd., suite 630
Newport Beach, Ca. 92660
tel. 714-851-1550

In addition to the general mutliple vitamins and minerals above, most clients also take supplemental fish oil (MaxEPA), L-Carnitine, and Coenzyme Q-10. The dosages of these supplements vary with each individual, depending upon their age, blood profile, blood lipid levels and disease manifestations. As a general rule, however, MaxEPA is taken at six capsules (6 gms.) per day, 3 in the morning and 3 at night. L-Carnitine is taken at 500 milligrams twice a day, and Coenzyme Q-10 is supplemented at 60 milligrams per day.

Depending upon the individual characteristics, a variety of other supplements are utilized accordingly. For instance, Pantothenic Acid, at 500 milligrams twice a day is often given a therapeutic trial for men and women who complain of excessive fatigue for which no specific reason can be found.

Patients with diabetes, high blood pressure, and heart disease are routinely given 300 to 900 milligrams of magnesium in addition to the 500 milligrams of magnesium contained in the Forward formula. In many cases, magnesium injections are used to rapidly replenish depleted magnesium stores.

Niacin is often used in various doses as an aid in lowering the blood-cholesterol level.

Literature on how various nutrients can be used to treat health problems is expanding rapidly. Therefore, individuals receive a specialized program tailored to their needs and problems.

For more information on the vitamins and minerals that are used by the Institute, please contact our office at the address above.

Now that you are armed with a healthy supplement program, let's put in the final piece of the puzzle—an exercise regimen.

—8—

Physical Fitness: A Key to Better Blood Chemistry

People who are sluggish and who rarely exercise can improve some aspects of their blood profiles by incorporating regular body movement into their daily routine. Weight-bearing exercises (walking, running, jogging, bicycling), for instance, will increase calcium production in the bones, preventing osteoporosis. Atherosclerosis can be avoided by increased exercise, which will prevent blood fats from depositing calcified cholesterol plaque along arterial walls, thereby blocking the artery and preventing red blood cells from making necessary oxygen deliveries. It's also possible to overcome some damage of cholesterol plaque by widening the arteries with a regular exercise program, thus providing extra space for blood flow so that more oxygen can be delivered throughout the body. Diabetics find it easier to control blood sugar (glucose) when they add regular exercise to their regimen, and those who suffer from high blood pressure can also benefit from increased movement of the body, which will cause better control and normalization of hypertension. Last but not least, regular exercise improves the function of the heart muscle and its ability to perform oxygen interchange with the lungs and to stimulate optimal blood flow throughout the body.

There are basically two types of physical exercise. There is anaerobic (also called isometric) and aerobic (also called isotonic). Each has a role in strengthening the muscle structure of the body and in providing better heart-muscle capability, lung capacity, and oxygen delivery.

113

ANAEROBIC/ISOMETRIC EXERCISE

This is the type of exercise in which the muscle groups expend a considerable amount of energy over a short period of time, such as lifting a heavy weight. It gets the name "anaerobic" because the massive amount of energy required to lift a heavy weight is done in bursts of energy that require more oxygen than the heart and blood vessels are able to deliver at that instant. You cannot continue an anaerobic exercise for a long period of time. For instance, if you were hoisting a hundred pounds over your head, you perhaps could do this one or two times, and that's it. Likewise, if you were trying to "chin yourself," or pull up on a horizontal bar, elevating your chin above the bar, you would not be able to keep up this kind of activity much longer than a few minutes.

Such short bursts of energy are called isometric because the muscle fibers are contracting against an immovable or only slowly movable object. Although the hundred-pound weight is moved, it is moved only a short distance with great effort.

True isometric exercise requires the participant to push with considerable effort against an immovable bar or object. Deliberate effort can be made to exercise specific muscles in the body using an almost stationary method of exertion.

AEROBIC/ISOTONIC EXERCISE

Aerobic activity is the muscle work or contraction that is sustained for a considerable length of time. For instance, in bicycling, you can push the pedal down sixty times per minute, which means you would depress the pedal with one leg 1,800 times in thirty minutes. During aerobic exercise, the heart delivers the appropriate amount of oxygen necesary to sustain the repetitive contraction of the large muscle group, enabling you to keep up this kind of activity for much longer periods of time.

It is also called isotonic because the activity and muscle contraction it generates can turn an easily movable object, such as a bicycle pedal, or can use your whole body in movement, as when you walk, jog, or swim.

STRENGTH AND CONDITIONING

A visit to an exercise facility often combines both anaerobic and aerobic movement. Exercise physiologists often refer to such regular exercise as giving a strength and conditioning benefit. Conditioning exercises would be the aerobic variety, involving body movement such as walking, jogging, and aerobic dancing. Working with weights or machines that isolate the various muscle groups of the body is strength or anaerobic exercise. The combination of strength and conditioning is important, as the musculature of our bodies supports our skeleton, determines to a great extent our posture, and helps to maintain body tone, while increased oxygen delivery helps to lower risk factors in the blood.

If you are not the type to go to a gym on a regular basis, and if you plan to choose only one exercise, such as walking, that's fine. Aerobic exercise like walking conditions the heart, blood vessels, and skeletal muscles to be able to maintain such activity for long periods of time. There are many benefits to be gained from selecting such an exercise to do on a regular basis:

- *Weight control.* Aerobic-conditioning exercises are necessary for any weight-loss or weight-maintenance program. Walking, swimming, or jogging on a regular basis will to a great extent burn fat and will facilitate the body's ability to burn fat and clear the blood of excess fat.
- *Resetting the metabolic thermometer.* The facilitated burning of fat will rev up your metabolism and accelerate weight loss. If you were to walk briskly for twenty minutes, you would burn about 8 to 10 calories per minute over what you would burn in the resting state. This would add up to 160 to 200 calories during the twenty-minute exercise session. If this were the only attribute of exercise for caloric expenditure, it might not be worth the effort as an aid to losing weight. However, the metabolic effects of a twenty-minute walk do not end when the walk does—regular aerobic exercise resets the "metabolic thermometer," helping the body to burn fat and other sources of fuel at a higher rate throughout the day.

If you plan to add aerobic exercise to your routine, and if you have been sedentary most of your life (particularly if you are a male over age forty), be sure to have heart and stress tests first. Also, be sure to start slowly and add a bit more distance every day.

- *Cardiovascular conditioning.* Aerobic exercise improves cardiovascular conditioning in several ways. First, the heart becomes stronger and more efficient with aerobic exercise training. An important characteristic of good aerobic conditioning is a slower resting heartbeat. In the sedentary population, the resting heartbeat will average about 65 to 80. In those participating in aerobic conditioning programs, the resting heartbeat will average 45 to 65. The reason for this slower heart rate is that a stronger, more efficient heart requires less beats per minute in the resting state to deliver the same amount of oxygen.

• *Oxygen extraction.* Another benefit of aerobic conditioning is an improved capacity to extract oxygen from blood. This can be demonstrated in both the resting state and the exercising state. Blood flowing through the heart and large muscles contains a set amount of oxygen. Not all of this oxygen is extracted from the blood before it is returned to the heart and lungs, but in a conditioned individual, a much greater percentage of oxygen is extracted than in a sedentary person.

This ability to extract oxygen from the blood in a more efficient way can be lifesaving if someone were to experience a heart attack. It is generally believed that heart attacks are less frequent in aerobically conditioned men and women, but those that do occur are less severe and more than likely not fatal, as compared to heart-attack statistics of unconditioned people.

• *Collateral circulation.* Whenever fat and cholesterol begin to block an artery, the body responds by building "collateral arteries" that will bypass the danger point. Exercise is the only activity that can facilitate adding such natural bypasses of blocked vessels. By exercising the heart muscle and putting it under controlled stress on a regular basis, the heart is stimulated to produce collateral circulation more rapidly. This ability is of utmost importance when an artery gets blocked.

• *Mood elevation.* Right now you may feel good—optimistic, calm, and with a general sense of well-being. On the other hand, you could be depressed. You may be fatigued, pessimistic, irritable, or you may have a generally reduced interest or enthusiasm for life. You may have lost your interest in sex, or even the interest you have in maintaining good friendships. Aerobic exercise can improve all of that. Besides reducing the risk of a heart attack, helping control diabetes, preventing osteoporosis, and helping you to maintain normal weight, aerobic exercise will make you feel better because it stimulates adrenal hormone such as epinephrine and noradrenaline—powerful mood elevators. Exercise also stimulates beta-endorphin hormones, which are the most active mood elevators of all. If you need to get rid of "blue days," start an exercise program that will help you to enjoy life again.

THE EXERCISE PRESCRIPTION

The exercise prescription should have four components: type of exercise, duration of exercise, exercise pulse rate to achieve, and frequency of exercise per week. For the majority of patients evaluated, a prescription will be written for either walking or brisk walking. For some, the prescription will be for swimming, bicycling, aerobic dancing, or other forms of aerobic conditioning. For instance, Bill, a fifty-two-year-old insurance executive, received a prescription that required him to walk briskly (which for Bill would mean a walking pace of four miles per hour, or one mile in fifteen minutes), for a half hour per day, reaching a pulse rate of 130, exercising five times per week.

You can achieve excellent results in aerobic conditioning by following such a prescription. Even better to achieve optimal results (if your doctor approves) would be to set a goal to walk briskly two miles a day, five days a week, which equals ten miles a week. By following this regimen for thirty minutes each day, you can walk 520 miles a year. Remember to build up your capacity gradually if this is your goal. It will improve your blood profile, oxygen delivery, and your general good health!

THE EXERCISE STRESS TEST

Before you begin the exercise program outlined above, consult your physician, who will likely give you a fitness test. Perhaps the most valuable test assessing the health of the heart and physical conditioning is the exercise stress test. This test allows the physician to observe the function of the heart under the stress of increased aerobic activity. Again, it's an important test to take before embarking on a rigorous exercise program.

When you walk briskly, jog, or ride a bicycle, there is an increased and dramatic demand for blood and oxygen in the large muscles. At maximum activity, a well-trained athlete can increase the blood flow circulating through his body by tenfold, or one thousand percent. The heart delivers this acceleration by increasing the number of beats per minute and the amount of blood pumped by each heartbeat.

During the exercise stress test, a patient is hooked up to an electrocardiograph machine while walking briskly on a treadmill or riding a stationary bicycle. The physician carefully watches a monitor that shows the electrical activity in the heart. The pulse rate of the heart, as displayed on the stress-test machine, is monitored by a trained technician or nurse who regularly measures the blood pressure.

If the heart is to increase its workload by tenfold, it requires an increase in blood and oxygen to make it possible. The blood and oxygen that are delivered to the heart muscle flow through the coronary arteries of the heart. If these arteries have blockages of fat and cholesterol, the amount of blood that is available to the heart muscle is decreased. When the heart tries to increase its workload without sufficient blood and oxygen to support this extra effort, the electrocardiogram of the heart changes. This change in the electrocardiogram is called a depressed ST segment.

Below is the configuration of the normal electrocardiogram. This electrical pattern consists of a "P wave" representing the initiation of electrical activity in the atrium of the heart. This is followed by a "QRS," the large spike of electrical activity generated by the large and powerful ventricles of the heart. Then there is a pause, represented as the "ST segment," and this is followed by the "T wave," which represents repolarization of the left ventricle, making it ready for another heartbeat.

When there are blockages in the heart arteries, an insufficient amount of blood and oxygen is available for the increased demand of activity. This causes some characteristic changes in the normal EKG (electrocardiogram) pattern of the exercising heart.

The most significant change is an "ST segment depression." A lack of oxygen causes the ST segment to depress below the baseline prior to the repolarization of the T wave.

On the EKG strip, the amount and type of ST segment depression can be measured. If the ST segment depression is slightly depressed but has an

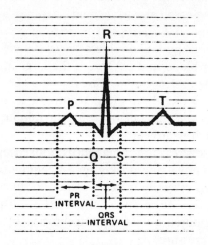

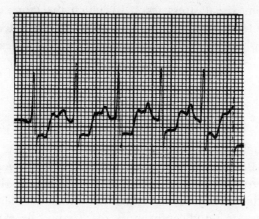

upsloping characteristic, it is not considered to be indicative of significant blockages in the coronary arteries. "This is called a "J point depression."

If the ST segment is horizontal in the depressed state or even downward sloping, it does indicate inadequate heart blood flow.

Generally, the degree of ST segment depression correlates with the degree of blockages in the coronary artery. A markedly positive stress test for coronary-artery blockage would have an ST segment depression horizontal or down-sloping and measuring two or more millimeters from the baseline.

Pulse Rate During the Stress Test

The stress test is also indicative of the pulse rate achieved by the patient with vigorous activity. An estimate of the maximum pulse rate a person can achieve at times of maximum exercise is equal to 220 minus the patient's age. For instance, if you are a forty-year-old man and are running through the jungle with five cannibal savages in hot pursuit, you would be expected to reach a pulse rate of 180 (220 minus 40) beats per minute. This, however, is only an estimate. The actual maximum pulse rate of any individual can only be assessed with a "maximum exercise test," which increases amounts of exercise on the treadmill until the patient cannot keep up. This is rarely done and then only on extremely well-conditioned athletes. What is generally

119

done is a "submaximal stress test," in which the target pulse rate to be achieved by the test is 85 percent of the maximum calculated pulse rate. This means that the physician would stop the test in the forty-year-old man when he reached a pulse rate of 85 percent of 180 (180 × .85), or 153 beats per minute.

Blood Pressure During the Stress Test

Another valuable measurement of the stress test is the behavior of the blood pressure. Both the systolic (upper) and diastolic (lower) blood pressure elevate in a normal individual undergoing a stress test. The systolic blood pressure characteristically elevates much more than the diastolic blood pressure. If both elevate significantly more than would be expected, then the patient would have exercise-induced hypertension.

If the blood pressure falls during the stress test, the test should be stopped immediately because it indicates that the left ventricle (the ventricle of the heart muscle responsible for delivering blood to the entire body) is beginning to ail, a serious finding.

CARDIAC MEDICATIONS AND EXERCISE

Ironically, some of the most common medications given to patients with heart disease and angina pectoris (chest pain from heart disease) weaken the heart and reduce its ability to pump extra blood needed during exercise.

Beta-blocker medications, such as Inderal, Tenormin, Corgard, and Lopressor, effectively block the response of the heart and other tissues to the stimulating hormone epinephrine produced in the adrenal gland. An elevation of this hormone causes the heart to beat faster and more strongly, as well as increasing the blood pressure in the arteries by causing their muscle walls to contract. Epinephrine also increases the amount of oxygen required by the functioning heart and other muscles.

These beta-blocker medications block the sensitivity of the heart and other muscles to epinephrine, thus reducing the ability of the heart to increase both its pulse and strength of contraction in response to exercise. However, they do have a role in the treatment of patients with heart disease, reducing the amount of oxygen required by the heart to function and often preventing angina pectoris and heart attacks.

Another group of drugs, newer than beta-blockers, are called calcium channel blockers. They include Cardizem, Isoptin, and Procardia. The calcium channel blockers alter the influx of calcium into the muscle cells of the heart and blood vessels, reducing the heart's ability to increase its rate and strength during exercise.

Heart patients taking beta-blockers and calcium channel blockers characteristically have very low resting pulse rates, as well as low pulse rates in response to exercise. Often a brisk walk by patients on these medications does not stimulate a pulse higher than 75 to 90, when in normal individuals the same degree of activity would result in a pulse rate of 115 to 130.

It's important for patients taking these drugs to know that they significantly alter the response they will have to the exercise stress test. Often, they cannot elevate their pulse while on the treadmill. Even more significant, the blood pressure of patients taking these medications frequently falls in response to exercise. Physicians are aware that a falling blood pressure in response to exercise in patients taking these drugs does not have the same dangerous connotation that it would in patients not taking these drugs.

(For more information about blood warnings for heart disease, read chapter 10.)

Physical Conditioning

In addition to demonstrating the presence of heart problems, the exercise stress test is a good indication of cardiovascular and physical conditioning. Patients who are well-conditioned can exercise at a very high "MET level" and have very high "VO2" consumption.

The MET level (metabolic equivalent) is represented as a multiple of the energy the body requires, or is consuming, while sitting quietly in a chair. This metabolic equivalent equals one. If you are walking at 3 miles per hour, up a five-degree grade, you are expending 5.5 times the amount of energy required to sit quietly in a chair. Therefore, the MET level is equal to 5.5. If you begin to jog slowly at 5 miles per hour up the same grade, the MET level jumps to 10.

There are numerous protocols for the stress test that gradually increase the effort by increasing the speed or the inclination of the treadmill. On the exercise bicycle, the MET level is raised by increasing the resistance of the bicycle, or the resistance mode on the bicycle wheel. Trained athletes can often exercise at a MET level of 15 to 20 for considerable lengths of time. The average population exercises at MET levels of 5 to 10. For someone in excellent condition, exercising at a MET level of 7 results in only a modest increase in pulse rate, while someone in poor condition approaches maximum pulse rate at the same MET level.

VO2 Max

The VO2 max is a measurement, often calculated, of the maximum oxygen intake the individual can reach with exercise. Like the pulse rate, there is a gradual decline in the maximum oxygen intake with age. The maximum oxygen intake can be estimated by the patient's weight, the MET level achieved during exercise, and the pulse rate. Or, the VO2 max can be measured. The individual on the treadmill wears a mask, creating a large reservoir that captures the air expired from the lungs. This expired air is then analyzed for the amount of carbon dioxide and residual oxygen present. VO2 max is a valuable statistic for cardiovascular conditioning because it measures the amount of oxygen that is delivered and consumed by the body.

At the Whitaker Wellness Institute, the stress test is used not only to screen patients for the presence or absence of heart disease, but also to serve as a basis for an exercise presecription. Exercise, along with diet and a sound program of vitamin and mineral supplements, is a key factor in improving your blood profile and your general good health.

——9——

Cancer Prevention Through Healthy Blood Profile

Cancer, even though it is not the most deadly degenerative disease in this country (heart disease kills roughly three times more people per year than cancer), is the most feared. This fear stems from the suffering brought on by cancer and the treatment currently used for cancer.

At present there is no test routinely used that is a reliable indicator of cancer. However, there are several tests that are used to indicate progression, regression, or successful treatment of cancer that has already been diagonsed. It is from these tests that a predictive test will likely come in the future.

Early cancer detection may not yet be a reality, but today the best method of preventing cancer is to increase your general health, strengthening your immune system and forming a *barrier* to the development of cancer.

Even in the absence of a specific blood test predicting cancer, we know enough about the relationship between many cancers and various aspects of lifestyle to prevent cancer. In summary, the key cancer preventers seem to be:

- Low-fat diet
- Increased dietary fiber
- Plenty of deep green and yellow vegetables for beta-carotene
- Aerobic exercise
- Maintenance of ideal weight

- Nutritional supplements that include vitamins C and E, selenium, and beta-carotene
- Avoiding known carcinogens

WHAT IS CANCER?

Cancer is actually many different diseases with many causes, ranging from leukemia—abnormal numbers and forms of immature white blood cells in circulation—to skin cancer, which itself can be a single lesion or one that has metastasized throughout the body. Basically, however, cancer can be defined as tissue cells that lack a controlled growth pattern, thus invading and destroying normal tissue cells.

Cancer generally develops from normal cells. Sometime during its life a cell may sustain some damage. This damage may not be enough to kill the cell, but enough to change the cell in such a way that it begins to multiply without control. At this stage the immune system has broken down, allowing the cell to multiply, and the single cancer cell becomes the cancer disease. Our approach to cancer prevention is to strengthen the immune system via lifestyle changes that involve diet, exercise, and vitamins and minerals, so that the body can destroy such cells before they multiply.

Often the damage occurs several years before the cell begins to spread as cancer. In the 1950s, women were sometimes given the drug Diethylstilbestrol during the first trimester of pregnancy. The female offspring of these women had a very high incidence of cancer of the vagina in the late teens. Also in the fifties, doctors would sometimes x-ray the thymus gland in young children if it was thought to be enlarged. Twenty years later, these patients, as adults, developed cancer of the thyroid.

There are many things in life that can damge the cell and cause cancer to blossom. Aside from possible genetic factors, cancer researchers have found cancer to be caused by what they term "carcinogens." Carcinogens are divided into two major groups: *initiators,* or cancer-causing agents that damage a cell's DNA (genetic material), leaving cells prone to becoming cancerous; and *promoters,* or agents that support the cell's transformation from normal to cancerous over a period of time. It has been said that just because a cell has been damaged by an initiator doesn't mean it will become cancerous. It is the promoter that usually enables a cell to aberrate.

This initiation/promotion model of carcinogenesis is not perfect, however. In fact, it is difficult to label a substance a carcinogen because circumstances dictate carcinogenicity. It would be safe to say that in some instances a potential carcinogen acts as an initiator and in some as a promoter, depending upon the conditions. It's a "which came first, the chicken or the egg" situation.

One study found, for example, that high-fat diets exert an effect on tumorigenesis (tumor growth) when administered *after* the carcinogenic agent, thus acting as the promoter. *(Progr. Biochem. Pharmacol.,* Vol. 10: pp. 308–353, 1975.)

However, another study revealed that fats can act as the initiator of cancer in four ways. First, increased fat in the blood alters cell-membrance fluidity, decreasing "metabolic cooperation" between cells to such an extent that the cells become isolated from the normal checks and balances of the body and can proceed along abnormal metabolic pathways characteristic of cancer. Second, excessive dietary fat alters production of prostaglandins from linoleic acid. These potent, hormonelike substances have a powerful effect on the body's immune system, and the production shift brought on by fat alters this system in a negative way. Third, dietary fat alters various hormones in the body that then abnormally stimulate their target organs. For instance, dietary fat abnormally increases the hormone prolactin and some of the estrogen hormones in women, which partially explains the association of excessive dietary fat and cancer of the breast, the target organ of these hormones. Fourth, dietary fat alters the bacteria in the colon, which is thought to play a big role in the onset of colon cancer. (*Gynecology and Obstetrics*, pp. 558–561, 1986.)

DIET AND CANCER

We probably don't even know all of the possible mechanisms by which environmental factors, diet, and nutrition are related to the etiology of cancer. However, some possible origins of cancer are:

• Carcinogens in food (e.g., chemicals added in production or naturally occurring chemicals formed during growth such as those found in the nodules of legumes).

• Oxidant damage to cells; lack of antioxidant substances in the diet. (These will be discussed in detail later in the areas of fats and prevention.)

• Excessive intake of certain nutrients (e.g., animal fat, fats in general, iron, alcohol, vitamins).

• Altered solubility of nutrients and/or carcinogens caused by dietary factors (e.g., fiber).

• Altered enteric bacterial population of the colon (e.g., excessive dietary fat causes a more dangerous form of bacteria to dominate the colon. Antibiotics and low fiber diets also cause bacterial population changes).

• Chromosome damage cause by nutrient deficiency.

• Abnormal repair of chromosome damage (e.g., caused by nutritional deficiencies).

• Altered metabolism of hormones (e.g., in obesity).

• Impaired immunity to tumor cells and viruses (e.g., caused by ingestion of chemicals or the deficiency of necessary nutrients).

• Genetic "susceptibility" plus dietary factors (*Contemporary Nutrition,* Vol. 5, No. 12, December, 1980.)

It is obvious that many of these mechanisms intertwine. Many share, for example, nutritional deficiencies as their common denominator.

KNOWN CARCINOGENS IN FOOD

The following known carcinogens have been observed as both initiators and promoters, depending upon the circumstances. It is insignificant in most cases to worry about whether the carcinogen initiated the cancer or promoted it. It would be wise to consider, rather, that regardless of how each carcinogen functions, all are "armed and dangerous."

We will begin with chemicals because they are truly the *least* of our concern! Even though carcinogenic properties of frequently ingested chemicals generate a lot of publicity, the actual danger of most chemicals causing cancer compared to the carcinogenic properties of high-fat, animal-protein foods is often negligible. The typical reaction to the numerous reports of chemical carcinogens is, "Well, everything causes cancer." However, a low-fat, high-fiber diet with supplementation of various antioxidant nutrients such as vitamins C, E, and A (beta-carotene) can go a long way to strengthen the immune system against any carcinogenic change. Therefore, the best defense against cancer is first to eat the foods that protect against it, then to avoid the specific chemicals that have been found to promote it.

SACCHARIN Various chemicals have been in the news as being "carcinogenic." One very famous one is the artificial sweetener, saccharin. Is it carcinogenic? From what we've learned so far, we'd have to say, maybe yes, maybe no. Again, it depends on the circumstances. Some considerations might be: How much is being used? How well does the consumer's immunity function? What

126

other potential carcinogenic materials are being simultaneously consumed? According to *The New England Journal of Medicine,*

> The diabetic whose perception of the quality of life is markedly improved by the availability of a sweet drink and the middle-aged man whose use of one packet of artificial sweetener per day in his morning coffee is important to his self-image can be assured that the excess risk of bladder cancer from such practices, if present at all, is quite small and little cause for concern. On the other hand, the general patterns of use of artificial sweeteners in this country are troublesome. The heaviest use is by women in the childbearing years. There has also been in increase in use among children, who are receiving much higher doses (per kilogram of body weight) than adults.

The article goes on to warn against "excessive use," such as four or more artificialy sweetened drinks per day, especially by children, teens, and pregnant women. (*The New England Journal of Medicine,* Vol. 302, No. 10: pp. 573–574, March 6, 1980)

This is all to reiterate, of course, that carcinogens are not definitive little villains with a scarlet C written on them. A person must exercise wisdom in this matter.

ALCOHOL, CAFFEINE, AND TOBACCO Wherever upper-alimentary-tract cancer is found, the key risk factors have been associated with chewing of opium tars, pickled and salted foods in the diet, smoking or chewing tobacco, along with deficiencies in protective nutrient factors.

Smoking has been associated with lung cancer.

Stomach cancer has been associated with a high consumption of dried, salted, pickled, and smoked foods, along with low intake of protective foods like fresh vegetables and fruits.

Pancreas cancer has been associated with tobacco use, possibly alcohol, the use of refined carbohydrates like white bread, and carcinogens produced from deep-frying or broiling of meat or fish.

All of these are complicated by an extraordinarily high-fat diet, and all are alleviated by protective factors such as high intake of beta-carotene and other protective foods that will be discussed later in more detail. *(Gynecology and Obstetrics,* pp. 558–561, 1986.)

Just be aware that chemicals in excess, or in any amount to a susceptible host, can initiate cancer. In fact, we could write an encyclopedia about potential chemical carcinogens. Furthermore, our worry over exposure to such chemicals as food additives is out of proportion. We ingest these substances in parts per million. What has been found to be *more* important regarding the epidemic of cancer in the world today is not chemicals at all but our dietary fat consumption, which we ingest in grams per day! For this reason, we will focus the remainder of this chapter on this area and on prevention.

Fats

POLYUNSATURATED FATS It has been proven that the development of some (possibly all) tumors is dependent upon the availability of essential fatty acids. Polyunsaturated fats, in particular, have been shown to accelerate the growth of tumors in rodents. However, once the requirement for the essential fatty acids had been met in this experiment, all digestible fats were equally effective in enhancing tumor growth. *(Contemporary Nutrition,* Vol. 11, No. 4; 1986.)

What do polyunsaturated fatty acids do? In experimental animals it was found that they contribute to breast tumors by inhibiting cellular communication, with aberrant prostaglandin production, and by their "cocarcinogenic action" (i.e., "feeding the tumor"). *(Eur. J. Cancer Clin. Oncol,* Vol. 23, No. 4: pp. 407–410, 1987.) Additionally, when polyunsaturated fats inside the body undergo partial oxidation (peroxidation), they split incompletely into what are known as free radical particles. These are extremely reactive, often combining undesirably with other substances or attacking cell membranes. (Maurice Finkel, *Fresh Hope with New Cancer Treatments,* Prentice–Hall, 1984, p. 67.)

Polyunsatured fats? you say. Aren't these the "good guys" I buy in the bottle from the health store marked, "unrefined, cold-processed, no cholesterol"?

Yes, that's them. Dr. Myron Winick, professor of nutrition at Columbia University's College of Physicians and Surgeons has stated, "A pattern has developed that is seen more in developed countries than undeveloped countries," of which "the strongest correlation is related to the intake of total fat: The higher the intake, the greater the incidence of colon and breast cancer." (Robert Steyer, "Cancer Probers Placing More Emphasis on Nutrition," *Sunday Star-Ledger,* Section One: p. 79, May 27, 1979.) However, monosaturated fats, such as olive oil, appear to be much less dangerous.

Dr. Winick isn't just spouting opinions, either; his statement is well-founded.

128

Numerous studies indicate that the worldwide distribution of breast cancer, for instance, clearly indicates that this disease (like most types of human malignancy) is correlated to the intake of dietary fat.

Consider the following:

- In Thailand, the intake of dietary fat is approximately 25 grams per day, and the death rate from breast cancer is less than one in 100,000.
- In Spain, the intake of dietary fat is approximately 100 grams per day, and the death rate from breast cancer is approximately 8 in 100,000.
- In the United States, the intake of dietary fat is approximately 150 grams per day, and the death rate from breast cancer is approximately 22 in 100,000.
- In Denmark, the intake of dietary fat is approximately 155 grams per day and the death rate from breast cancer is approximately 23 in 100,000.

In fact, when the fat intakes and death rates from breast cancer of countries are represented graphically, it is clear that the higher the fat intake, the greater the incidence of breast-cancer deaths. *(Federation Proceedings*, Vol. 35, No. 6; pp. 1309–1315, May 1, 1979.)

MONOUNSATURATED FATS A very interesting finding in regards to monoun-saturated fats (e.g., olive oil) is that this type of fatty acid *lacks tumor-promoting properties. (Gynecology and Obstetrics*, pp. 558–561, 1986.) This would explain why Mediterranean countries, which consume a high-fat diet, show lower breast-cancer rates than would be expected. It is because the fats they consume are primarily monounsaturated.

How Much Fat Is Too Much?

Interestingly, it has been found in studies with mice that tumor incidence increased when the dietary level of fat exceeded 15 percent. (Cancer Research, Vol. 35, November, 1975, pp. 3292–3300.) Conversely, it has been predicted that if postmenopausal women with stage II breast cancer were able to stick to a 15 percent or less fat diet for five years, their disease-free survival rate would be far greater than in women who maintain the 40 percent fat diet typical of most Americans.(*Gynecology and Obstetrics*, 1986, pp. 558–561.) This is of special interest to us now because we have set a goal of lowering our current 40 percent of calories as fat to no more than 20 percent. The studies encourage our efforts!

It has also been found that transplanted tumors in rats and mice can be significantly retarded by feeding the animals diets free of cholesterol or free of cholesterol and fat. In this same study, as in the study mentioned previously, a chart demonstrates that there is a significant association between fat consumption and deaths from breast cancer in women.

PREVENTING CANCER WITH GOOD NUTRITION

Epidemiological studies as well as laboratory observations have established many nutrient factors that show anticarcinogenic properties. From an article on nutrients and cancer prevention, we quote:

Nutrients that act as anticarcinogens to prevent cancer initiation or growth may function by:
- picking up active forms of cancer-initiating componds (carcinogens) and preventing them from functioning to initiate cancer cell growth;
- alteration of the body's defense systems;
- inhibition of tumor initiation via alteration of cell metabolism;
- prevention of gene activation and cellular proliferation by tumor promoters;
- inhibition of cancer progression once it has been initiated by the alteration of cell differentiation. (*Journal of American Diet.* pp. 505–510, April, 1986.)

The chart on page 131 shows the initiators and promoters associated with various human cancers, and the protective elements associated with these same cancers.

GREEN AND YELLOW VEGETABLES AND FRUITS Emphasizing dark green and deep yellow fresh vegetables and fruits increases your consumption of vitamins A and C and fiber. The reason these three nutrients are anticarcinogenic is discussed under their individual headings. Examples of deep green and yellow vegetables and fruits are: carrots, spinach, other greens, sweet potatoes, peaches, apricots, and oranges. Juicy fruits, of all kinds, however, are rich sources of vitamin C, and possibly A as well.

VITAMIN A OR BETA-CAROTENE When we speak of vitamin A we mean preformed vitamin A found only in animal-source foods, such as fish-liver oils. A primarily vegetarian diet supplies vitamin A in its precursory form as beta-

NUTRITIONAL FACTORS INVOLVED IN HUMAN CANCERS

TYPE OF CANCER	Potential Initiators	Potential Promoters	Protective Nutrients
Esophagus, oral cavity	Tobacco, opium tars, salting and pickling	Alcohol, low intake of micronutrients	Green and yellow vegetables, fruits high in vitamins A, C, and E
Stomach	Dried, salted, pickled, smoked fish and foods, high nitrate levels in food and water	Salt, low intake of fruits, and vegetables, and low intake of vitamin C	Increased intake of fresh vegetables and fruits; Vitamins C and E
Pancreas	Tobacco? Fried meats and fish?	Alcohol? Coffee? High dietary fat intake	Fresh fruits and vegetables, low-fat diet
Large bowel	Carcinogens formed in fried or broiled meat and fish (heterocyclic amines)	High level of dietary fat, bile acids	Cereal bran fiber, cruciferous vegetables, selenium, calcium. Olive oil? Fish oils? Exercise?
Large bowel, Rectum	??	Alcohol?	Fiber?
Breast	Fried meats and fish?	High dietary fat intake; hormone imbalance?	Low-fat diet, olive oil, fish oils
Endometrium	??	Postmenopausal estrogen intake, high-fat diet, obesity	Low-fat diet, olive oil, fish oils
Ovary	??	High-fat diet	Low-fat diet
Prostate	??	High-fat diet	Low-fat diet, adequate selenium

carotene. The body manufactures the vitamin A it needs from beta-carotene. Because excess A can be toxic, beta-carotene, which is richly supplied by consuming dark green and yellow vegetables and fruits, is a safer source.

Beta-carotene as Vitamin A is needed so that cells lining the tissues of the body can be varied according to their functions, not abnormally alike or indistinguishable. Scientists call this the "normal differentiation of epithelial cells." This function of vitamin A has been known for years, but researchers have only recently connected beta-carotene deficiency with the cancer process.

Beta-carotene itself has long been thought to be simply a precursor of vitamin A and virtually useless until transformed into vitamin A. However, recently scientists have observed that carotenoids themselves can act as "free radical traps," which means they are efficient anticarcinogens. Four hundred carotenoids have been isolated from nature, with only about fifty demonstrating biological activity, of which beta-carotene is the most plentiful and active. (*Vitamin Nutrition Information Service*, Vol. 1, No.1.)

VITAMIN C Epidemiological studies reveal that vitamin C may lower the risk of cancer, particularly in the esophagus and stomach. This revelation is consistent with studies done on experimental animals that show that vitamin C is effective in blocking the transformation of nitrites into carcinogenic nitrosamines. *(Contemporary Nutrition,* Vol. 10, No. 10, October; 1985.) Nitrites, in the form of potassium and sodium nitrite, are most commonly used as a color fixative in cured meats like hot dogs, bologna, and bacon. When ingested they combine with natural stomach and food chemicals to form nitrosamines, powerful cancer-causing agents. (So if you must eat a hot dog, eat an orange with it!)

A study on cancer and vitamin C, using 100 patients with advanced stages of cancer and 1,000 similarly afflicted patients as the control group, found that, when given 10 grams of ascorbic acid daily, patients lived on the average over four times as long as the matched controls.

Vitamin-C therapy is also said to help normal tissues surrounding a malignant tumor resist infiltration by that tumor by strengthening the intercellular cement that binds the cells of the normal tissues together. *(Executive Health,* Vol. 16, No. 4; January, 1980.)

Preventing nitrites from forming carcinogenic nitrosamines and strengthening the intercellular cement of cells are two important functions of vitamin C. Perhaps there are many more we have yet to discover.

VITAMIN E Vitamins A, C, and E, in addition to selenium, all function as antioxidants working together to protect cell membranes from free radical–related damage. Vitamin E, along with vitamin C, inhibits the conversion of nitrites to nitrosamines in the stomach. Epidemiological studies show that even with less than optimal consumption, intake of vitamins A, E, and C results in a lower incidence of certain cancers. *(Vitamin E Research & Information Newsletter,* Vol. 1, No. 5; July, 1986.)

A research update from *The American Institute for Cancer Research Newsletter* states:

Vitamin E's most important function in our bodies is to prevent a highly destructive process called lipid peroxidation. Lipid peroxidation can destroy fragile cell membranes and generally wreak havoc to our cells' inner structures. This process can also change the cell's DNA (its genetic material), a necessary first step in the development of cancer.

Lipids, of course, are fats. A low-fat diet would be the ideal, but when fats *are* consumed, vitamin E should accompany them. Natural fats have a certain amount of vitamin E, but some researchers insist that supplementation is necessary to obtain an amount sufficient for potential benefits. (Ibid.)

CEREAL BRAN FIBER Fiber lowers the risk of colon cancer by speeding the time for undigested food to pass through your large bowel. This, of course, could limit exposure of your colon lining to cancer-producing chemicals. Some forms of fiber have the ability literally to absorb chemicals and fats, binding them into harmless waste matter and passing them out of the body before they can do any harm.

But if there were nothing "magical" about fiber, it is at least a very satisfying nutrient, giving a feeling of fullness. Also, fiberous foods are generally very low-fat foods, and therefore an excellent substitute for fattier, undesirable foods. Additionally, fiberous foods are almost always those foods that are rich sources of the anticarcinogenic nutrients vitamins A, C, and E, and minerals like selenium. In fact, as detrimental as fats are to the human state of wellness, fiber is essential. Perhaps nothing would be more beneficial to the world at large, and to the affluent populations in particular, than a simple avoidance of fats and an emphasis on fiber. Not only cancer, but virtually all diseases, would decrease dramatically.

CRUCIFEROUS VEGETABLES Certain vegetables in this family (cabbage, broccoli, brussels sprouts, kohlrabi, and cauliflower) may help prevent certain cancers from developing. Call them "antipromoters." This protective factor has been labeled a vitamin in the past, but current reports state that cruciferous vegetables contain "indole derivatives that act as enzyme inducers," which seem to inhibit carcinogenesis. (Ibid.)

SELENIUM Selenium, a micromineral, is found in minute amounts throughout the body tissues. It functions with vitamin E as an antioxidant, preventing cell damage from peroxidized (degraded) fats. A deficiency would be difficult to detect because vitamin E and some amino acids can substitute for selenium in some of its functions. Rich sources are fish and yeast, but grains grown on nondepleted soils are good sources as well. Generally speaking, high-protein foods contain a lot of selenium.

Of course, it is selenium's function as an antioxidant that protects cells from the damage fats can do and thereby protects the body against carcinogens.

CALCIUM We all know about the necessity of calcium for bone formation and maintenance. Lesser known is the need for calcium in nerve-message transmission, controlling heartbeats, muscle contractions, blood clotting, and activating many enzymes. However, in regard to the participation of calcium in anticarcinogenesis, it has been found that calcium may protect against colon-cancer development by binding fatty acid and bile acids, and also by reducing the rate of intestinal cell duplication. (*The New England Journal of Medicine*, Vol. 313, 1985, pp. 1381–1384.) Reducing bile acids within the colon reduces mutagens in stools, which are apparently produced by specific bacteria directly influenced by intestinal bile-acid levels. (J. H. Weisburger and E. L. Wynder, *Important Advances in Oncology*, Philadelphia: J. B. Lippincott, 1987.)

OLIVE OIL AND FISH OILS In experiments with animals, as well as in epidemiological observations, researchers have found that polyunsaturated fats are more effective promoters of breast cancer than even saturated fats, although it is ultimately the total-fat level that is significant. However, fish oils and olive oil *do not* have tumor-promoting effects in animal studies.

The reasons why some fats contribute to carcinogenesis and why some do not are not fully understood. In part the fatty acids themselves "feed cancer," and in part products generated during the metabolism of fats are involved. It is even suspected that the excess calories provided by fat may be directly involved. The research continues.

The above is not an exhaustive list of anticarcinogenic nutrients. For example, zinc has been cited in cancer avoidance, as have medium-chain triglycerides. In fact, anything that boosts immunity, acts as an antioxidant, eliminates bacteria, fungi, viruses, etc., or does not impart injury to the consumer could be anticarcinogenic.

EXERCISE Along with the development of agricultural techinques came the evolution of excessive meat eating. We produced more, we ate more. Simultaneously, man worked less vigorously for his daily bread, becoming more sedentary, even in leisure time. The result has been what can be called "overnutrition." Excessive amounts of cholesterol and nutrients—especially fats—increase levels of blood lipids, which adversely affect the arterial wall, and bile acids, which have been implicated in carcinogenesis. Of course this begins a snowball effect, where one bad thing leads to another, ending in diseases of every kind, including cancer.

— 10 —

Reversing Blood Warnings for Heart Disease

If you want to prevent a disease, prevent heart disease. Heart disease is by far the most serious disease afflicting the American population. It kills more people than cancer, diabetes, accidents, or all other causes of disease combined. It claims close to 3,000 lives per day, and is one of the worst epidemics in the history of man.

The first symptom of heart disease is often sudden death. Men and women die from this malady without any warning 44 percent of the time. No other disease acts like this. Cancer, diabetes, AIDS, and pneumonia all make themselves known far before the fatal outcome. They give both you and your physician a fighting chance to overcome the disease.

Dr. Jeremiah Stamler, chairman of the Department of Community Health and Preventive Medicine at Northwestern University Medical School and coordinator of the Multiple Risk Factor Intervention Trial (MRFIT), has been a vocal opponent of the complacency of most physicians regarding the total-cholesterol level.

The MRFIT study, in an effort to identify the major risk factors of heart disease, screened 356,222 men aged thirty-five to fifty-seven with no history of heart disease and followed them over a six-year period. There were over 7,000 heart attacks during that time, and the death rate from heart disease increased within each age group as the level of serum cholesterol increased.

Dr. Stamler pointed out that the total-cholesterol level is one of the most sensitive predictors of oncoming heart attack. It is both "graded" and "continuous." Graded means that as the cholesterol increases, the risk of heart disease increases proportionately. Continuous means that there is no particular "dangerous threshold" above which heart disease occurs.

This is contrary to the belief of many physicians, who consider cholesterol ranges in men up to 280 to be "normal," when indeed they were found to be indicative of significant risk.

For instance, in the forty to forty-four age group, men with cholesterol levels of 182 to 202 have a 77 percent higher death rate from heart disease when compared to men with cholesterol levels of 182 or lower. A group of men at the upper end of the scale, with blood-cholesterol levels measuring in excess of 263, have a 562 percent higher death rate from heart disease than the group with cholesterol levels of 182 or less.

As Dr. Stamler stated, "In every one of these groups, this relationship held consistently, systematically, and without contradiction, and in every one of them it was continuous, strong, and graded from the second 20 percent of serum cholesterol (182–202 milligrams per deciliter) on up." *(Medical Tribune, February 5, 1986, p. 3.)*

The serum blood total-cholesterol level is one of the most predictive measurements of impending heart disease.

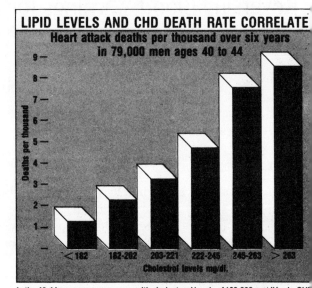

LIPID LEVELS AND CHD DEATH RATE CORRELATE

Heart attack deaths per thousand over six years in 79,000 men ages 40 to 44

Deaths per thousand / *Cholesterol levels mg/dl.*
(<182, 182-202, 203-221, 222-245, 246-263, >263)

In the 40-44 age group, even men with cholesterol levels of 182-202 mg/dl had a CHD death rate 77% higher than those with levels below 182, Dr. Stamler said.

The process of atherosclerosis (fat and cholesterol plugging arteries), which is the primary cause of heart attacks and heart disease in this country, progresses silently. You cannot feel it, nor do you know that it is happening until finally the artery blockages are so severe that heart attacks, often fatal, occur "out of the blue." Therefore, a program to prevent cardiovascular disease is the first order of business for most Americans. However, there are two other reasons for making heart-disease prevention the primary focus of your health maintenance program.

First, the specific blood warnings for heart disease are much clearer than the warnings for other diseases. For instance, blood-cholesterol level, blood pressure, cigarette smoking, and the absence of exercise can be statistically related to the risk of developing a heart attack. The blood warnings for other diseases also have predictive power, but they are not nearly so defined and mathematically reproducible as the blood warnings for heart disease.

Secondly, a vigorous program to eliminate the risk of cardiovasculaar disease encompasses appropriate diet, exercise, vitamin and mineral supplementation, and techniques to lower the blood pressure, all of which produce the state of "optimal health" for the participant and alter a variety of the blood measurements in a beneficial fashion. It is safe to say that for the majority of those who vigorously follow a program to prevent heart disease, their blood chemistries change in dramatic fashion—all for the good. In short, the more effective your program is at preventing heart disease, which means significantly altering the blood warnings for heart disease, the healthier you will become.

A corollary to this is that the healthier that you become, the better you feel, function, and enjoy life. A vigorous program to prevent heart disease also builds strong barriers against diabetes, obesity, and complications of high blood pressure, such as strokes. If an appropriate and vigorous program to prevent heart disease is maintained, the patient will have an ideal laboratory panel in all areas, as well as the ideal physical measurements, such as blood pressure, weight, and percent body fat.

CASE HISTORY

The power of a vigorous heart disease program is best illustrated by the experience of Mr. John O'Donnell. He was given the tools to save his life, and he did, and in the process his health and functioning were enhanced a thousandfold.

After graduating from college, John began to teach at the college level. At that time, his perceptions of the "good life" meant fancy restaurants and indulging regularly in his favorite wines and beers.

He began gaining weight while teaching college, but this was nothing compared to what was to come.

In high school he had been very active in athletics, playing on the football and basketball teams. He had always been thin and noted that his blood pressure had always been very low. We do not have available laboratory tests from that period, but one can only assume that at that time they were much better than after seven years of his "good life." After college he stopped exercising almost completely, which increased his tendency to gain weight.

He began a business career by buying and selling gold coins. Since this was more profitable than his teaching profession, he pursued the new career. As he continued in his success, his time became limited, with his exercise pattern becoming nonexistent. With affluence, he began to lose control over his lifestyle and health. Over a seven-year period he gained over one hundred pounds very slowly.

Blind to the Problem

John never saw that he had a problem. He would look at himself in the mirror, and that extra hundred pounds hanging from his bones just wouldn't register other than his thinking that he might be a "little" overweight.

Then one day in a drugstore he took his blood pressure and found it to be 165 over 105. This jolted him, as he had had low blood pressure throughout his entire life. He had heard Dr. Whitaker lecture about diet and exercise as tools to lower blood pressure and to prevent heart disease, and called the Whitaker Wellness Institute to enroll in a two-week program.

At that time, John was thirty-eight years old and had no overt disease, but he was literally riddled with indications of "impending" disease. His weight was obviously up, his blood pressure was elevated, and his blood panel revealed these findings

Cholesterol level 251
HDL Cholesterol 34
LDL Cholesterol 148
VLDL Cholesterol 69
Cholesterol: HDL ratio 7.4
Uric acid 8.2
Triglycerides 344
Glucose 90

Calculating John's Risk Level

By processing the known factors that elevate risk of heart disease, a computer program can calculate the risk of heart attack for an individual over an eight-year period. This information was gleaned from the Framingham studies over the last thirty years.

The Framingham Studies

The Framingham Studies are quite unique. They started right after World War II in Framingham, Massachusetts, and represent attempts by doctors at that time to isolate specific factors for assessing risk of heart disease. Close to 6,000 men in Framingham were recruited for the study. Their only obligation was to report to a study physician and have various tests made every six months to a year. No therapy was offered by the Framingham Study physicians.

At the time these men were recruited for the study, they had no known heart disease and were considered to be in good health. As they began to die from various diseases, the data collected on them over the years was assessed. It became apparent after ten to fifteen years that certain measurable factors in men without heart disease increased their risk of having a fatal heart attack.

It is from the Framingham Studies that the whole concept of "risk factor" (a measurable factor associated with varying risk of disease) was developed. The risk factors that surfaced almost immediately were blood-cholesterol level, blood pressure, and presence of cigarette smoking. In men who had high blood-cholesterol levels there was a definite increase in frequency of fatal and nonfatal heart attacks. The same was true for elevation in systolic blood pressure and the presence of cigarette smoking. Essentially, men who had higher blood-cholesterol levels, higher systolic blood pressures, and smoked, had a far greater risk of having fatal heart disease than men with low blood-cholesterol levels, low blood pressure, and who did not smoke. It was found that each "risk factor" acted independently. This meant that men with high blood pressure had a higher risk than men with low blood pressure. Men who smoked had a higher heart-disease risk than those who did not. Men with high blood-cholesterol levels had a greater heart-disease risk than those with low blood-cholesterol levels.

It also became apparent that an elevated blood-cholesterol level (above 150 milligrams per cubic centimeter) was essential for heart disease to occur,

141

regardless of the presence or absence of other risk factors. This meant that if the blood-cholesterol level was not elevated substantially above 150, then the presence of cigarette smoking, high blood pressure, or inactivity would *not* increase the risk of a heart attack.

As we learn more and more about the process of atherosclerosis, this observation begins to make sense. Cholesterol plugging requires elevated blood-cholesterol levels. In the presence of elevated blood-cholesterol levels, other factors such as high blood pressure, cigarette smoking, elevated uric acid, and elevated white blood cells accelerate the process. Without significantly elevated cholesterol levels, however, the process cannot occur. Therefore the presence of the other known risk factors cannot produce the cholesterol blockage in the arteries themselves.

At this stage, John certainly had enough cholesterol in his blood for atherosclerosis, so the other risk factors were working against him in a dangerous way. His calculated risk panel was not encouraging.

Summary of Cardiovascular Risk Factors: John O'Donnell

Age: 38	Sex: Male
Blood cholesterol: 251	HDL Cholesterol: 34
Systolic blood pressure: 150	Blood sugar: normal
Changes on EKG: None	Cigarettes: No
Overweight: Yes	Regular Exercise: No
Family history of heart disease: No	
Present risk of heart attack over next 8 years: 57 per 1000	Average Framingham risk for persons in this age range: 41 per 1000

Relative risk*: 1.39

*Relative risk is present risk divided by average Framingham risk.

At age thirty-eight, John had a 6 out of 100 chance of having a heart attack over the next eight years. This risk was about 40 percent higher the average risk of men his age in the Framingham studies.

In discussions with John, we asked him what his goals were. He said he wanted to lose one hundred pounds, essentially eliminate his risk of heart disease, regain his physical strength and endurance, and, in general, improve his health and sense of well-being.

The first order of business for John, and for preventing heart disease, is to lower the blood-cholesterol level. There are numerous drugs that can lower the blood-cholesterol level, but none of them should ever be used until the basic cause of mose elevated cholesterol levels is addressed—inappropriate diet.

For most Americans on their high-fat, high-animal-protein diet, 15 to 30 percent of the circulating cholesterol can be accounted for in the diet. Therefore, diet alone could be expected to lower John's cholesterol level to the 175–214 range. This could be expected simply by eliminating the rather substantial amounts of saturated fat and cholesterol he was consuming at the time of his initial interview. John was instructed to lay off the cheeses, eliminate egg yolks entirely, cut down substantially on red meats (particularly fatty ones), avoid the insidious salad dressings, particularly those that contain eggs or cheese, and to replace them with fruits, vegetables, grains, and pastas, with a concentration on vegetable foods that are low in saturated fats and contain no cholesterol.

A second dietary factor for control of cholesterol that was used by John was a consistent increase in dietary fiber, particularly pectin fibers found in fruits, as well as oat-bran fiber. These are water-soluble fibers and are the most effective dietary fibers for lowering the blood-cholesterol level. They absorb cholesterol in the intestinal tract and increase its excretion in the stool.

John was also put on multiple vitamins and minerals similar to the ones described in chapter 7, to ensure that his metabolic systems were saturated with the known and appropriate "coenzymes" (the major function of most micronutrients) for optimal metabolic function.

Exercise

We cannot overemphasize the importance of physical exercise in the prevention of cardiovascular disease. As pointed out in chapter 8, regular aerobic exercise strengthens the heart muscle, lowers the resting pulse rate indicating more efficient heart function, enhances the extraction of oxygen from the blood, and facilitates the development of collateral circulation that, by creating additional channels of blood, naturally bypasses areas of blockage.

When John first started his exercise program, this formerly well-trained athlete could hardly endure a brisk walk, owing to excessive obesity and poor condition. But walk he did, and his walking increased. After one year he was jogging for forty-five minutes per day. After a year and a half John was able to run a mile in five minutes. This represented tens of thousands of percent improvement in his physical conditioning and capacity.

John's blood pressure fell rapidly to very safe ranges. The reasons for this drop in blood pressure (which have been discussed elsewhere) will be mentioned here in review.

The fat in his diet was reduced substantially, which has been shown to lower blood pressure. Sodium, or table salt, was also reduced in conjunction with an increase in potassium intake from substantial amounts of vegetables and fruits and potassium-based salt substitute, such as Nu-Salt, Nosalt, or Morton salt substitute. His vitamin-and-mineral program included additional calcium, and his proteins were derived now primarily from vegetable sources, both of which have been shown to lower blood pressure. His dramatic increase in physical activity and physical conditioning also had a beneficial effect upon his blood pressure.

John's Education

An integral part of this health program was educating John to understand what was necessary, why it was necessary, and what benefits he would derive from his efforts. He became quite aware of the important of his laboratory values, and copies of all tests done on him were given to him to compare with previous measurements. Thus John had a sense of participating in, if not guiding, his own program with the help of physicians.

The open sharing of laboratory information with patients and clients is essential to any program that is going to be successful in preventing cardiovascular disease or improving health.

As John continued to become healthier, his enthusiasm for life increased: to say that he "felt better" is an understatement. But the real proof of the benefits he received from his program was demonstrated by the change in his blood profile and his calculated reduction in risk of having a heart attack.

At age thirty-nine, after one year on the program of diet, exercise, and nutritional supplements, his risk-factor profile was submitted to the computer again with the following results.

Summary of Cardiovascular Risk Factors: John O'Donnell

Age: 39

Blood cholesterol: 113

Systolic blood pressure: 110

Changes on EKG: None

Overweight: No

Family history of heart disease: No

Sex: Male

HDL cholesterol: 60

Blood sugar: Normal

Cigarettes: No

Regular exercise: Yes

Present risk of heart attack over
the next 8 years: 3 per 1000

Average Framingham risk for
persons in this age range: 41
per 1000

Relative risk: .073

In one year, his risk of having a heart attack had been reduced by 95 percent! When he first started the program, his chances of having a heart attack were about 140 percent the average risk in Framingham. After one year, his risk had dropped to only 7 percent of the average Framingham risk. And he felt much better to boot.

The menu and recipe sections that follow in this book will put you on the best preventive medicine diet possible. It will help you to get your own blood profile into normal ranges so you can enjoy the rest of your life in good health.

— 11 —

Your Game Plan and Menus

As with anything you want to accomplish, you must have a plan. If you do not know where you are going, you won't go anywhere.

Optimal health is simple to define, easy to document, and the tools are at your fingertips. The difficulty everyone has with healthy living is that what must be done, must be done regularly. Optimal health is far easier to maintain in an experimental animal whose food and activity level can be strictly controlled than in an intelligent human being who makes his or her own choices.

Regularity requires discipline and organization. As frightening as those two words are to most people, the secret to staying on track is to "put it in black and white." First decide what you want to accomplish and write it down. Then decide what is necessary to reach your goal and write that down. Then do what you write down. It's that simple.

MAKE YOUR GOALS SOMETHING YOU CAN ACCOMPLISH AND GIVE YOURSELF TIME TO ACHIEVE THEM

It is one thing to set high standards and quite another to shoot for the impossible. Make your goals something that you know you can accomplish over a reasonable period of time. For instance, you may be thirty-five pounds overweight with a variety of abnormal blood measurements and high blood pressure.

You attempt to lose the entire thirty-five pounds and straighten everything

147

else out in two weeks. You fail. Now you have the perfect excuse to give up the program. It doesn't work!

The successful way to be successful is to make reasonable goals, accomplish them, and make more. Add successes to success.

WHEN MAKING YOUR PROGRESS CHARTS, USE THE "KIS" PRINCIPLE: KEEP IT SIMPLE

There is no need to be elaborate. If you accomplish the key goals, everything else will fall into place. Start with the basics.

Body Measurements: What Do You Want to Look Like?

	PRESENT	WEEK 1	WEEK 2	WEEK 3	WEEK 4	WEEK n*	OPTIMUM
Weight							
Waist Measurement (measured at the navel)							
Hip Measurement							
Body-fat percentage							

n is the number of weeks you plan to take to accomplish your goals.

Physiological Measurements: What Do You Want to Be Like?
(For these you will need your physician's assistance)

	PRESENT	(6 WEEK INTERVALS)	OPTIMUM
Blood pressure			
Blood measurements (after 10-hour overnight fast)			
Cholesterol			>200mg%
HDL cholesterol			<40mg%
HDL: cholesterol ratio			Male >3.43
			Female >3.2
Triglycerides			>200mg%
Glucose			>100mg%
Uric acid			>5mg%
BUN			>15mg%

HOW YOU ARE GOING TO GET THERE

Organize Your Diet

The trick to changing your diet is to decide what you are going to eat before you eat it, and then to eat it.

Plan your meals. Write down what you are going to eat. Then eat it.

Weekly Menu Planner

	Breakfast	Lunch	Dinner	Snack
Monday				
Tuesday				
Wednesday				
Thursday				
Friday				
Saturday				
Sunday				

Decide On an Exercise

What do you like to do? What can you do? What can you easily incorporate into your daily life? In short, what *are* you going to do?

- Walking
- Brisk walking
- Stationary bicycle (excellent for bad weather)
- Swimming
- Aerobic dancing
- Treadmill in the home (excellent for bad weather)

Find the time to do your exercise for at least thirty minutes, five days a week.

Determine how high your pulse should be. This is best done with a stress test, but a good training pulse can be derived by the following formula:
Training Pulse = 220 − AGE × .70 (or .85 if you are more vigorous)
Measure your pulse before you start (BPR), at your peak exercise level (PPR), and after five minutes of recovery (RPR).

Record your progress.

Day*	Pulse Rates						
	EXERCISE	BPR	PPR	RPR	TIME	DISTANCE	COMMENTS
Monday							
Tuesday							
Wednesday							
Thursday							
Friday							
Saturday							
Sunday							

*You should not exercise vigorously every day. Five days a week is optimal, or exercise five harder days with two easier days in the week.

Vitamin and Mineral Supplements

Put yourself on a good vitamin-and-mineral supplement program, and stay with it. The program used here at the Whitaker Wellness Institute is outlined, and if you want more information about it, please contact us at 440 MacArthur Boulevard, Newport Beach, CA 92660.

Usually it is best to take supplements with meals and, for convenience, the morning and evening meals are best.

SOME TRICKS TO IMPROVE THE HEALTH PROFILE

To Lower Blood Cholesterol

- Lose weight
- Increase the fiber in your diet with pectin fiber supplements, oat-bran muffins, two apples a day
- Niacin supplements. Though it is not a prescription item, the dose of niacin necessary to lower blood cholesterol is substantial and should be monitored by a physician experienced in its use
- L-Carnitine, 1,000 milligrams per day

To Lower Triglycerides

- Exercise aerobically five days a week
- Lose weight
- MaxEPA supplements of fish oil, three to five per meal
- Niacin (see above)
- Increase the fiber in your diet (see above)
- Decrease alcohol and sugar consumption
- L-Carnitine, 1,000 milligrams per day

To Lower Blood Pressure

- Eat more potassium-rich foods *every day:* fresh fruits and vegetables
- Supplement with calcium, 1,000 milligrams per day
- Supplement with magnesium, 500 milligrams per day
- Exercise aerobically for a half hour five days a week
- Drink 8 to 10 ounces of fresh vegetable juice per day. The juice should be made at home or bought from a health-food store. *It should not be a canned variety with added salt!*
- Increase garlic and onion consumption
- Use a potassium-based "salt substitute" regularly at meal times. (If

you have significant kidney damage, or are on a potassium-restricted diet, check with your physican before doing any of these suggestions.)

INTRODUCING THE MENUS

It is said that blood is the river of life. Just as modern people have polluted the rivers of our nations, so many people have polluted their bloodstreams by making a habit of poor food choices. When blood tests are performed, the results can give clues to impending debilitating degenerative disease. These tests can reveal lurking dangers long before a medical calamity happens. Poor test results put you on notice to do something about specific findings that can be reversed with change of diet. Later blood tests can confirm that you have been successful at averting trouble.

By now you understand the importance of having your blood evaluted and of changing any factor that is above or below normal ranges. But just as blood is the river of life, food is one of the pleasures of existence. No one wants to change eating habits only to lose all the foods he or she loves. The good news is that you can enjoy wonderful meals despite all restrictions. The recipes in this book were created to prove the point that you can eat well and be well at the same time.

There is an art to implementing a new way of eating. First, take a look at your food shelves. If they are filled with canned and packaged prepared products, appraise how they will fit in with your wiser lifestyle. Those that are high in fat, salt, and sugar should be given away.

What you will need is a supply of brown rice, barley, dried beans, salt-free and sugar-free whole-grain cereals, pasta in all shapes and sizes, unsalted canned tomatoes and tomato sauce, unsweetened canned fruit, a variety of dried herbs and spices, olive oil and other unsaturated vegetable oils, and cider or tarragon vinegars. Water-processed decaffeinated coffee or a variety of herbal teas would also be welcome.

Keep a supply of unbleached and whole-wheat flours in small quantities if you plan to bake. Honey, brown sugar, and molasses may be used in small amounts for sweetening. Dried raisins and frozen apple juice concentrate will also be used in recipes for sweetening and flavor.

The refrigerator should be stocked with eggs (for egg whites), fresh vegetables, and fresh fruit. Skim milk, grated Parmesan cheese, and low-fat cheeses such as sapsago, one-percent-fat cottage cheese, skim-milk ricotta cheese, and plain nonfat yogurt should also be available. Fish and poultry should be purchased as needed.

Whenever you buy bread, be sure that it is a whole-grain, whole-wheat, or rye variety. Get the higest concentration of B vitamins and fiber that you can for the money.

As you can readily see, you will be saving money when food marketing because you will have no need of high-priced prefabricated food products with this diet program. Our goal is to keep it simple and keep it delicious, matching the expertise of experienced chefs who know that straightforward cooking with exquisite seasoning wins applause every time.

As you read the recipes, notice that you will need some nonstick cookware—skillets in several sizes, loaf pans, and cookie sheets. You also might want a nonstick muffin tin, although you can use paper baking liners with a regular muffin tin if you prefer.

It's wise to have several heavy saucepans and a large soup pot. The heavier the metal, the more even the heat and the less chance you will have of burning the food. Several nonstick casseroles of various sizes will also come in handy as you prepare one-dish baked meals.

No modern kitchen should be without an electric mixer (a hand mixer will do) and an electric blender or electric food processor (or both). A microwave oven is helpful for baking potatoes and apples at the last minute, for heating frozen or fresh vegetables, and for reheating leftovers. Some people claim that they are also good for cooking meals from scratch, but their lack of browning ability and need for frequent turning are drawbacks.

Naturally, you will need the basic equipment of every cook—such things as wooden spoons, rubber spatulas, ladles, measuring cups and spoons, a vegetable peeler, and a good can opener. The most important thing to remember when equipping a kitchen is to be able to reach for the tool you need to make the cooking easy and fun.

We know that you are involved in a busy life and cannot dedicate a lot of time to cooking. You will find that the recipes in this book respect your need for fast and healthy fare. Every recipe includes a nutritional analysis for each serving so you know exactly what you are eating. A thirty-day menu program is included to take the guesswork out of planning meals. Refer to the cholesterol and calorie charts at the back of the book if you need further help in choosing complementary foods that hold to the theory of smart eating.

You may have to relearn cooking techniques. These recipes omit frying, sautéing, and other fat-filled cholesterol builders. You will find that recipe directions for this book are simple to follow. As you put the salt shaker away, you may become the best short-order chef you know as you enter the fascinating world of seasoning with herbs and spices.

Thirty-Day Menu Program to Reverse Blood Warnings

What could be easier than following a well-balanced menu plan for each day, enabling you to make sure that you are getting all the protein, carbohydrates, fat, vitamins, minerals, and fiber that you need to function well. Following are one month of such menus based on an approximate intake of 1,600 calories a day. This is a maintenance diet for good health which takes into consideration that you will be including some form of exercise each day.

Extremely active people may add extra complex carbohydrates to these menus for a total of 1,800 to 2,000 calories a day. Do this in the form of another starch and another vegetable or two and fruit. Also, extra fiber and calories may be added to any meal by adding a slice of whole-grain bread at 50 calories a slice.

If you desire to have a lower caloric intake for weight loss, you can easily determine what extra items to omit until you have reached optimal weight. Giving up the mid-afternoon and bedtime snacks can cut about 300 calories per day—the best way to cut down the calories of these menus. It is generally considered to be unwise to go below a 1,200-calorie intake each day if you want to be sure you get a good balance of nutrients—it's better to step up your exercise to burn off excess calories.

For purposes of simplification, we have rounded out the number of calories for some foods. For instance, we count each slice of bread as 50 calories and each unspecified piece of fruit as 100 calories. Where recipes are given in the book, you will find the name of the dish followed by an asterisk, and exact nutritional-analysis calories per portion will be used.

The menus are intended as a guideline to give you the feel of how to pattern a day's food. There will be times when you will be away from home and unable to follow a menu exactly. Just make a similar substitution, keeping in mind that all meat, poultry, and fish portions should be no more than four ounces and should not be cooked or served with any form of fat.

If you need a snack at bedtime, make it a cupful of fat-free, salt-free popcorn or two graham crackers and a half cup of fruit juice.

When eating in a restaurant, don't be embarrassed to specify that the waiter instruct the cook to omit all fat, salt, and sugar from your food. Order foods that can be broiled to order. Avoid anything that will come from a steam table—it is generally salted and buttered to stay for hours. Watch out for soups in restaurants as well. They are most often seasoned with a heavy handful of salt. When dining in a Chinese restaurant, be sure to ask that monosodium glutamate be left out of your cooked-to-order dish. Chinese chefs can do wonders with bits of ginger and garlic to make up for the lack of salt. Chefs in Italian restaurants are perfectly capable of making a fresh tomato sauce, sometimes with fresh basil leaves if you are lucky.

Fast-food restaurants pose the greatest problem because of their fixed menus. Most of them have salad bars, however, and it is possible in some to order a baked potato. The trick with these is to limit the salad dressing to one tablespoon drizzled over the top (otherwise it's possible to add 400 fat-filled calories per ladle of dressing), and be sure that you order the potato without butter. If all else fails, order the smallest chicken or fish sandwich on the menu.

Whether at a restaurant or at home, whenever possible be sure to have a large mixed vegetable salad with one tablespoon of an olive-oil dressing. This will give you extra fiber at little caloric cost, while giving you the beneficial HDL cholesterol of olive oil.

These menus are provided so you can see how to pattern a day's meals to add up to 1,600 calories of low-fat, high-complex-carbohydrate, adequate-protein dining. There may be times when you want to make substitutions. Plain broiled or baked chicken may be substituted for any chicken or turkey dish. Plain broiled or baked fish may be substituted for any fish dish. Any pasta dish can be replaced with a one-cup portion of pasta topped with a plain tomato sauce. Most vegetables are interchangeable. If you have any doubts, consult the general calorie list in the back of the book.

When a fruit snack is mentioned, you may choose any piece of fresh fruit. When using canned fruit, be sure to purchase only the unsweetened or "packed in natural juice, no sugar added" kind.

Any slice of whole-grain bread is interchangeable with rye bread, pumpernickel bread, or a variety of high-fiber breads. All recipes for breads and muffins in this book are freezable. It is suggested that you bake each type once and freeze the rest in one-portion Ziploc bags so it will be easy to thaw out just what you need each day.

Any whole-grain cereal is interchangeable with any other cereal that is low in sodium, sugar, and unnecessary additives. Hot cooked oatmeal is exchangeable with any other cooked whole-grain cereal.

We use only low-fat or skim-milk dairy products. That way you get the calcium you need but not the fat. Read cheese labels carefully to determine the fat content.

As you can see, the attitude toward food in this book is of pleasure, satiety, and as a tool to improve your health. We hope you enjoy every meal of it!

Day One Menus

BREAKFAST	CALORIES
½ cup fresh strawberries, on	25
*Cottage Cheese Pancakes**	131
1 slice whole grain toast, with	50
½ teaspoon honey	10
Decaf or herb tea	0

LUNCH	
*Baked Noodles and Broccoli**	304
1 slice rye bread	50
Lettuce and tomato salad	40
½ cup unsweetened fruit	100
Decaf or herb tea	0

MID-AFTERNOON SNACK	
1 apple	100

DINNER	
*Curried Split Pea Soup**	61
*Broiled Flounder Parmesan**	249
½ cup cooked brown rice	100
1 cup cooked broccoli	40
Mixed green salad	10
1 tablespoon olive oil	100
1 tablespoon tarragon vinegar	2
*Prune Apricot Compote**	81
Decaf or herb tea	0

BEDTIME SNACK	
2 graham crackers	55
½ cup grapefruit juice	50

	Total	1608

Day Two Menus

BREAKFAST	CALORIES
1 cup orange juice	100
1 cup cooked oatmeal, with	150
¼ cup skim milk	25
Decaf or herb tea	0

LUNCH	
*Stuffed Baked Manicotti**	240
*Alfalfa Sprout Salad**	102
½ cup unsweetened fruit	100
Decaf or herb tea	0

MID-AFTERNOON SNACK	
1 fruit	100

DINNER	
*Potato Soup**	60
*Shish Kebab**	231
½ cup cooked brown rice	100
*Carrot Slaw**	38
1 slice rye bread	50
*Poached Pear**	122
Decaf or herb tea	0

BEDTIME SNACK	
2 cups popped corn	100
½ cup apple juice	60

	Total	1588

*Asterisk indicates that recipe, with caloric and nutritional information, appears in Part II, p. 171.

Day Three Menus

BREAKFAST	CALORIES
Tofu Banana Shake*	247
1 bagel, with	120
2 tablespoons 1% fat cottage cheese	20
Decaf or herb tea	0

LUNCH	
Vegetable Pasta Casserole*	268
Waldorf Banana Sprout Salad*	144
1 slice whole grain bread	50
Decaf or herb tea	0

MID-AFTERNOON SNACK	
1 fruit	100

DINNER	
Gazpacho*	43
Chicken Stroganoff*	215
1 baked potato, with	100
2 tablespoons plain nonfat yogurt	30
1 slice whole grain bread	50
Romaine salad	10
1 tablespoon Salt-Free Italian Dressing*	60
Nutty Carob Drop*	38
Decaf or herb tea	0

BEDTIME SNACK	
2 graham crackers	55
½ cup fruit juice	50
Total	1600

Day Four Menus

BREAKFAST	CALORIES
1 fruit	100
2 biscuits shredded wheat cereal, with	180
½ cup skim milk	45
Decaf or herb tea	0

LUNCH	
½ cup tomato juice	25
Creole Lentils*	222
Wheat Germ Slaw*	53
1 slice rye bread	50
½ cup unsweetened applesauce	50
Decaf or herb tea	0

MID-AFTERNOON SNACK	
1 fruit	100

DINNER	
Cream of Cucumber Soup*	30
Sole Rolls with Vegetable Sauce*	268
Baked Stuffed Butternut Squash*	119
Green salad	10
1 tablespoon Tofu Yogurt Dressing*	28
1 slice whole grain bread	50
Carrot Cookie*	75
Decaf or herb tea	0

BEDTIME SNACK	
1 cup Munch Bowl*	138
½ cup fruit juice	50
Total	1593

157

Day Five Menus

BREAKFAST	CALORIES
½ grapefruit	50
2 slices Cinnamon French Toast*	158
Decaf or herb tea	0

LUNCH	
Spaghetti with Tomato/Cucumber Sauce*	277
Romaine lettuce	10
1 tablespoon olive oil	100
1 tablespoon cider vinegar	2
1 slice rye bread	50
½ cup unsweetened fruit	100
Decaf or herb tea	0

MID-AFTERNOON SNACK	
1 fruit	100

DINNER	
Celery Pastina Soup*	89
Chicken Paprikash*	196
1 cup cooked brown rice	200
Spinach Mushroom Salad*	45
1 slice whole grain bread	50
Orange Sherbet*	76
Decaf or herb tea	0

BEDTIME SNACK	
2 graham crackers	55
½ cup grapefruit juice	50
Total	1608

Day Six Menus

BREAKFAST	CALORIES
½ cup orange juice	50
½ cup bran cereal, with	130
½ cup skim milk, and	45
½ sliced banana	45
Decaf or herb tea	0

LUNCH	
Apple Raisin Noodle Pudding*	216
Endive and Chickpea Yogurt Salad*	74
1 slice whole grain bread	50
½ cup unsweetened fruit	100
Decaf or herb tea	0

MID-AFTERNOON SNACK	
1 fruit	100

DINNER	
Black Bean Soup*	99
Monkfish in Mushroom Cream Sauce*	243
½ cup cooked brown rice	100
½ cup cooked brussels sprouts	30
Romaine lettuce	10
1 tablespoon Cucumber Dill Salad Dressing*	5
1 slice rye bread	50
Banana Orange Amandine*	133
Decaf or herb tea	0

BEDTIME SNACK	
1 cup popped corn	50
½ cup fruit juice	50
Total	1574

Day Seven Menus

BREAKFAST	CALORIES
½ cup fresh berries	25
*Banana Pancakes**	120
½ bagel, with	60
2 tablespoons 1% low fat cottage cheese	20
Decaf or herb tea	0

LUNCH	
½ cup tomato juice	22
*Baked Macaroni and Cottage Cheese**	260
*High C Salad**	46
1 slice rye bread	50
½ cup unsweetened fruit	100
Decaf or herb tea	0

MID-AFTERNOON SNACK	
1 fruit	100

DINNER	
*Barley Bean Soup**	78
*Chicken Stew**	285
Baked potato	100
2 tablespoons plain nonfat yogurt	30
*Tomatoes Vinaigrette**	56
*Oatmeal Raisin Muffin**	157
Decaf or herb tea	0

BEDTIME SNACK	
1 cup popped corn	50
½ cup grapefruit juice	50
Total	1609

Day Eight Menus

BREAKFAST	CALORIES
1 sliced orange	70
*Oatmeal Granola,** with	155
½ cup skim milk, and	45
½ sliced banana	45
Decaf or herb tea	0

LUNCH	
*Vegetable Soup**	26
2 servings *Kasha Tabbouli**	204
1 slice *Raisin Honey Rye Bread**	138
½ cup unsweetened fruit	100
Decaf or herb tea	0

MID-AFTERNOON SNACK	
1 fruit	100

DINNER	
¼ cantaloupe	30
*Broiled Lemon Flounder and Tomato**	260
1 boiled potato	90
*Cole Slaw with Roquefort Dressing**	39
½ cup cooked green peas	60
1 slice rye bread	50
1 *Carrot Raisin Date Cookie**	34
Decaf or herb tea	0

BEDTIME SNACK	
2 cups popped corn	100
½ cup fruit juice	50
Total	1596

Day Nine Menus

BREAKFAST	CALORIES
½ grapefruit	45
Egg White Cheese Omelet,* on	86
1 slice whole grain toast	50
Decaf or herb tea	0

LUNCH	
Linguine with White Clam Sauce*	300
Lettuce and tomato salad	40
1 tablespoon olive oil	100
1 tablespoon tarragon vinegar	2
1 slice whole-grain bread	50
½ cup unsweetened fruit	100
Decaf or herb tea	0

MID-AFTERNOON SNACK	
1 fruit	100

DINNER	
½ cup tomato juice	25
Broiled Turkey Rosemary*	213
Brown Rice Espanol*	125
Spinach Salad*	56
1 slice whole grain bread	50
Poached Pears*	122
Decaf or herb tea	0

BEDTIME SNACK	
2 graham carckers	55
½ cup unsweetened pineapple juice	50
Total	1569

Day Ten Menus

BREAKFAST	CALORIES
½ cup juice	50
½ cup bran cereal, with	130
½ cup skim milk, and	45
½ sliced banana	45
½ bagel, with	60
2 tablespoons 1% lowfat cottage cheese	20
Decaf or herb tea	0

LUNCH	
Lima Barley Soup*	102
Yolkless Spinach Frittata*	64
Baked potato	90
1 slice rye bread	50
Unsweetened fruit	100
Decaf or herb tea	0

MID-AFTERNOON SNACK	
1 apple	100

DINNER	
½ cup tomato juice	25
Crudites and Dip*	39
Stuffed Baked Red Snapper*	268
½ cup cooked brown rice	100
Collards Parmesan*	98
Date and Nut Muffin*	93
Decaf or herb tea	0

BEDTIME SNACK	
1 cup Munch Bowl*	138
½ cup fruit juice	50
Total	1567

Day Eleven Menus

BREAKFAST	CALORIES
½ cup orange juice	50
1 cup cooked oatmeal, with	150
¼ cup skim milk, and	25
1 tablespoon raisins	30
Decaf or herb tea	0

LUNCH	
Vegetable Soup*	26
Macaroni Stuffed Eggplant*	134
1 cup cooked broccoli	40
1 tomato, sliced	30
1 slice whole wheat bread	50
½ cup unsweetened fruit	100
Decaf or herb tea	0

MID-AFTERNOON SNACK	
1 fruit	100

DINNER	
Baked Chicken and Pineapple*	290
Baked sweet potato	155
½ cup cooked green beans	15
Whole Wheat Soda Bread*	118
Romaine lettuce salad	15
Tofu Yogurt Dressing*	28
Broiled Honeyed Bananas*	124
Decaf or herb tea	0

BEDTIME SNACK	
1 cup popped corn	50
½ cup apple juice	60
Total	1590

Day Twelve Menus

BREAKFAST	CALORIES
½ cup juice	50
Oatmeal Raisin Pancakes*, with	145
½ cup unsweetened applesauce	100
Decaf or herb tea	0

LUNCH	
Zucchini Lasagna*	142
Baked Lima Beans*	34
Tomatoes Vinaigrette*	56
1 slice whole grain bread	50
½ cup unsweetened fruit	100
Decaf or herb tea	0

MID-AFTERNOON SNACK	
1 fruit	100

DINNER	
Barley Bean Soup*	78
Halibut Mousse*	230
1 cup cooked broccoli	40
Mashed Potato Puff*	102
Carrot Slaw*	38
1 slice rye bread	50
Baked Apple with Lemon Raisin Topping*	144
Decaf or herb tea	0

BEDTIME SNACK	
2 graham crackers	55
½ cup apple juice	60
Total	1574

Day Thirteen Menus

BREAKFAST	CALORIES
1 sliced orange	70
½ cup 1% low fat cottage cheese	90
1 bagel	120
Decaf or herb tea	0

LUNCH	
Stuffed Eggplant*	87
Romaine lettuce	10
Sliced tomato	30
1 tablespoon olive oil	100
1 tablespoon cider vinegar	2
1 slice whole grain bread	50
½ cup unsweetened fruit	100
Decaf or herb tea	0

MID-AFTERNOON SNACK	
1 fruit	100

DINNER	
½ cup tomato juice	25
Zesty Turkey Loaf*	181
Lima Corn Casserole*	160
½ baked acorn squash	50
Cole Slaw with Roquefort Dressing*	39
1 slice rye bread	50
Apple Carob Brownie*	129
Decaf or herb tea	0

BEDTIME SNACK	
1 cup Munch Bowl*	138
½ cup grapefruit juice	50
Total	1581

Day Fourteen Menus

BREAKFAST	CALORIES
½ cup juice	50
½ cup bran cereal, with	130
½ cup skim milk, and	45
½ sliced banana	45
Decaf or herb tea	0

LUNCH	
1 cup Curried Split Pea Soup*	61
2 servings Spinach Cheese Soufflé*	88
High C Salad*	46
1 slice whole grain bread	50
½ cup unsweetened fruit	100
Decaf or herb tea	0

MID-AFTERNOON SNACK	
1 fruit	100

DINNER	
Gazpacho*	43
Poached Salmon Veronique*	225
Orange Rice*	132
½ cup cooked carrots	20
Lettuce salad	20
Salt-Free Italian Dressing*	60
1 slice whole grain bread	50
1 Honey Oatmeal Bar*	156
Decaf or herb tea	0

BEDTIME SNACK	
2 cups popped corn	100
½ cup fruit juice	50
Total	1571

Day Fifteen Menus

BREAKFAST	CALORIES
½ cup fresh strawberries, on	25
Cottage Cheese Pancakes*	131
1 slice whole grain toast	50
½ teaspoon honey	10
Decaf or herb tea	0

LUNCH	
Potato Soup*	60
Pasta Bow Ties with Yogurt Mushroom Sauce*	193
1 grated carrot, with	20
1 tablespoon raisins, on	30
Lettuce	10
1 tablespoon Tomato Juice Salad Dressing*	3
1 slice whole grain bread	50
½ cup unsweetened fruit	100
Decaf or herb tea	0

MID-AFTERNOON SNACK	
1 fruit	100

DINNER	
½ cup tomato juice	25
Oven-Fried Lemon Chicken*	278
1 baked sweet potato	155
½ cup cooked peas	60
Spinach Cauliflower Salad*	29
1 slice whole grain bread	50
Poached Apples*	86
Decaf or herb tea	0

BEDTIME SNACK	
2 graham crackers	55
½ cup fruit juice	50
Total	**1570**

Day Sixteen Menus

BREAKFAST	CALORIES
½ cup orange juice	50
Apricots and Grains*	149
¼ cup skim milk	25
Decaf or herb tea	0

LUNCH	
Baked Noodles and Broccoli*	304
Spinach Mushroom Salad*	45
1 slice pumpernickel bread	50
½ cup unsweetened fruit	100
Decaf or herb tea	0

MID-AFTERNOON SNACK	
1 apple	100

DINNER	
Tomato Rice Soup*	96
Herb Broiled Cornish Hens*	151
Carrot Stuffed Baked Potato*	103
Romaine lettuce	10
1 tablespoon olive oil	100
1 tablespoon cider vinegar	2
Ricotta Tofu Pudding*	128
Decaf or herb tea	0

BEDTIME SNACK	
2 cups popcorn	100
½ cup apple juice	60
Total	**1578**

Day Seventeen Menus

	CALORIES
BREAKFAST	
½ cup fruit juice	50
1 cup cooked oatmeal, with	150
¼ cup skim milk, and	25
1 tablespoon raisins	30
Decaf or herb tea	0
LUNCH	
1 cup chicken bouillon	50
Lasagna Florentine*	220
Carrot Slaw*	38
1 slice rye bread	50
½ cup unsweetened fruit	100
Decaf or herb tea	0
MID-AFTERNOON SNACK	
1 fruit	100
DINNER	
½ cup tomato juice	25
Linguine with Scallops*	384
Creole Green Beans*	23
1 slice whole grain bread	50
Fresh Fruit Delight*	51
Decaf or herb tea	0
BEDTIME SNACK	
1 cup *Munch Bowl*	138
½ cup grapefruit juice	50
Total	**1584**

Day Eighteen Menus

	CALORIES
BREAKFAST	
1 sliced banana	100
Oatmeal Granola*	155
½ cup skim milk	45
Decaf or herb tea	0
LUNCH	
Black Bean Soup*	99
2 servings Baked Kasha and Zucchini*	226
1 slice rye bread	50
Lettuce and tomato	40
½ cup unsweetened fruit	100
Decaf or herb tea	0
MID-AFTERNOON SNACK	
1 fruit	100
DINNER	
¼ canteloupe	30
Baked Spinach Balls*	209
1 cup cooked noodles	210
Cole Slaw with Roquefort Dressing*	39
1 slice whole wheat bread	50
Carrot Raisin Date Cookie*	34
Decaf or herb tea	0
BEDTIME SNACK	
1 cup popped corn	50
½ cup apple juice	60
Total	**1597**

Day Nineteen Menus

BREAKFAST	CALORIES
Tofu Banana Shake*	247
1 bagel, with	120
2 tablespoons 1% lowfat cottage cheese	20
Decaf or herb tea	0

LUNCH	
¼ cantaloupe	20
2 servings Eggplant Parmesan*	158
High C Salad*	46
1 slice rye bread	50
½ cup unsweetened fruit	100
Decaf or herb tea	0

MID-AFTERNOON SNACK	
1 fruit	100

DINNER	
Celery Pastina Soup*	89
Flounder with Broccoli Stuffing*	268
½ boiled potato	45
½ cup cooked carrots	20
Romaine lettuce	10
1 tablespoon Buttermilk Celery Seed Dressing*	8
1 slice whole grain bread	50
1 Poached Pear*	122
Decaf or herb tea	0

BEDTIME SNACK	
2 graham crackers	55
½ cup fruit juice	50
Total	**1578**

Day Twenty Menus

BREAKFAST	CALORIES
1 sliced orange	70
2 biscuits shredded wheat cereal, with	180
½ cup skim milk	45
Decaf or herb tea	0

LUNCH	
1 cup cooked spaghetti	210
½ cup Meatless Spaghetti Sauce*	28
Lettuce and cucumber salad	40
1 tablespoon olive oil	100
1 tablespoon cider vinegar	2
1 slice whole grain bread	50
½ cup unsweetened fruit	100
Decaf or herb tea	0

MID-AFTERNOON SNACK	
1 fruit	100

DINNER	
Tomato Rice Soup*	96
Roast Chicken with Prune Orange Stuffing*	178
1 cup cooked broccoli	40
1 baked potato	90
2 tablespoons nonfat yogurt	20
1 slice rye bread	50
½ grapefruit	50
Decaf or herb tea	0

BEDTIME SNACK	
2 cups popped corn	100
½ cup fruit juice	50
Total	**1599**

Day Twenty-one Menus

BREAKFAST	CALORIES
½ cup orange juice	50
2 slices *Cinnamon French Toast**, with	158
¼ cup unsweetened apple sauce	50
Decaf or herb tea	0

LUNCH	
*Fish Chowder**	163
*Brown Rice Cucumber Salad**	184
1 slice whole grain bread	50
½ cup unsweetened fruit	100
Decaf or herb tea	0

MID-AFTERNOON SNACK	
1 fruit	100

DINNER	
*Turkey Balls Ratatouille**	325
½ cup cooked noodles	105
Romaine lettuce	10
1 tablespoon *No-Oil Salad Dressing**	1
*Graham Carrot Muffin**	158
Decaf or herb tea	0

BEDTIME SNACK	
2 cups popped corn	100
½ cup fruit juice	50
Total	**1604**

Day Twenty-two Menus

BREAKFAST	CALORIES
½ cup orange juice	50
½ cup bran cereal, with	130
½ cup skim milk, and	45
½ sliced banana	45
Decaf or herb tea	0

LUNCH	
*Cabbage Soup**	46
*Rigatoni with Hot Chili Sauce**	220
Lettuce and tomato salad	40
1 tablespoon *Tofu Roquefort Dressing**	28
1 slice whole grain bread	50
½ cup unsweetened fruit	100
Decaf or herb tea	0

MID-AFTERNOON SNACK	
1 fruit	100

DINNER	
*Baked Cod Oreganata**	248
1 baked potato, with	90
2 tablespoons plain nonfat yogurt	30
*Spinach Mushroom Salad**	45
1 slice rye bread	50
½ cup *Orange Sherbet**	76
Decaf or herb tea	0

BEDTIME SNACK	
1 cup *Munch Bowl**	138
½ cup apple juice	60
Total	**1591**

Day Twenty-three Menus

BREAKFAST	CALORIES
½ grapefruit	50
Egg White Cheese Omelet*, on	86
1 slice whole grain toast	50
Decaf or herb tea	0

LUNCH

2 servings Baked Eggplant and To-matoes*	72
1 pita bread, stuffed with	150
Alfalfa Sprout Salad*	102
½ cup unsweetened fruit	100
Decaf or herb tea	0

MID-AFTERNOON SNACK

1 fruit	100

DINNER

Curried Split Pea Soup*	61
Sesame Chicken Kabobs*	261
½ cup cooked brown rice	100
1 cup cooked broccoli	40
Carrot Slaw*	38
Banana Raisin Bread*	123
Prune Apricot Compote*	81
Decaf or herb tea	0

BEDTIME SNACK

2 cups popped corn	100
1 cup fruit juice	100
Total	1613

Day Twenty-four Menus

BREAKFAST	CALORIES
½ cup fresh berries	25
Banana Pancakes*	120
½ bagel	60
Decaf or herb tea	0

LUNCH

Pasta with Shrimp Yogurt Sauce*	244
Spinach Sprout Salad*	88
1 slice whole grain bread	50
½ cup unsweetened fruit	100
Decaf or herb tea	0

MID-AFTERNOON SNACK

1 fruit	100

DINNER

Tomato Rice Soup*	96
Oatmeal Turkey Loaf*	166
1 baked sweet potato	155
½ cup cooked cauliflower	15
Cranberry Vegetable Mold*	70
1 slice rye bread	50
1 unsweetened baked apple	70
Decaf or herb tea	0

BEDTIME SNACK

1 cup Munch Bowl	138
½ cup fruit juice	50
Total	1597

Day Twenty-five Menus

BREAKFAST	CALORIES
1 sliced orange	70
½ cup bran cereal, with	130
½ cup skim milk, and	45
½ sliced banana	45
Decaf or herb tea	0

LUNCH	
Baked Macaroni and Spinach*	276
Romaine lettuce	10
1 tablespoon olive oil	100
1 tablespoon cider vinegar	2
1 slice whole grain bread	50
½ cup unsweetened fruit	100
Decaf or herb tea	0

MID-AFTERNOON SNACK	
1 fruit	100

DINNER	
½ cup tomato juice	25
Herb Stuffed Sole*	286
½ cup cooked brown rice	100
6 spears cooked asparagus	20
Herbed Cherry Tomatoes*	48
1 slice rye bread	50
Nutty Carob Drop*	38
Decaf or herb tea	0

BEDTIME SNACK	
2 graham crackers	55
½ cup fruit juice	50
	——
Total	1610

Day Twenty-six Menus

BREAKFAST	CALORIES
½ cup fruit juice	50
1 cup cooked oatmeal, with	150
¼ cup skim milk, and	25
1 tablespoon raisins	30
Decaf or herb tea	0

LUNCH	
2 servings Potato-Carrot Pancakes*	196
2 tablespoons plain nonfat yogurt, as topping	30
Broccoli Polonaise*	64
1 tomato, sliced	30
1 slice whole grain bread	50
½ cup unsweetened fruit	100
Decaf or herb tea	0

MID-AFTERNOON SNACK	
1 fruit	100

DINNER	
Black Bean Soup*	99
Poached Chicken Florentine*	228
½ cup cooked broad noodles	105
Lettuce salad	10
1 tablespoon Salt-Free Italian Dressing*	60
1 slice rye bread	50
Poached Pear*	122
Decaf or herb tea	0

BEDTIME SNACK	
1 cup popped corn	50
½ cup fruit juice	50
	——
Total	1604

Day Twenty-seven Menus

BREAKFAST	CALORIES
½ cup orange juice	50
½ cup bran cereal, with	130
½ cup skim milk, and	45
½ sliced banana	45
Decaf or herb tea	0

LUNCH	
½ cup tomato juice	25
2 servings *Baked Rice and Peas Amandine**	242
*Wheat Germ Slaw**	53
1 slice whole grain bread	50
½ cup unsweetened fruit	100
Decaf or herb tea	0

MID-AFTERNOON SNACK	
1 fruit	100

DINNER	
*Scallops Cacciatore on Pasta**	312
*Creamed Spinach**	35
Romaine lettuce	10
1 sliced tomato	30
1 tablespoon *Cucumber Dill Dressing**	5
1 *Oatmeal Raisin Muffin**	151
Decaf or herb tea	0

BEDTIME SNACK	
1 cup *Munch Bowl**	138
½ cup fruit juice	50
Total	1581

Day Twenty-eight Menus

BREAKFAST	CALORIES
½ grapefruit	50
½ cup 1% low fat cottage cheese	90
1 bagel	120
Decaf or herb tea	0

LUNCH	
*Gazpacho**	43
2 servings *Lima Corn Casserole**	300
Romaine lettuce	10
1 tablespoon olive oil	100
1 tablespoon cider vinegar	2
1 slice whole grain bread	50
½ cup unsweetened fruit	100
Decaf or herb tea	0

MID-AFTERNOON SNACK	
1 fruit	100

DINNER	
*Vegetable Soup**	26
*Chicken Mexicana**	287
1 cup cooked broccoli	40
*Pickled Cucumbers**	11
1 slice rye bread	50
*Carrot Cookie**	75
Decaf or herb tea	0

BEDTIME SNACK	
2 cups popped corn	100
½ cup fruit juice	50
Total	1604

Day Twenty-nine Menus

BREAKFAST	CALORIES
½ cup orange juice	50
2 biscuits shredded wheat cereal, with	180
½ cup skim milk, and	45
½ sliced banana	45
Decaf or herb tea	0

LUNCH	
½ cup tomato juice	25
Linguini with Vegetable Garlic Sauce*	267
Spinach Salad*	56
1 slice whole grain bread	50
½ cup unsweetened fruit	100
Decaf or herb tea	0

MID-AFTERNOON SNACK	
1 fruit	100

DINNER	
Cream of Cucumber Soup*	30
Flounder Creole*	225
½ cup cooked brown rice	100
Carrot Slaw*	38
1 slice rye bread	50
Banana Orange Amandine*	133
Decaf or herb tea	0

BEDTIME SNACK	
2 graham crackers	55
½ cup fruit juice	50
Total	**1599**

Day Thirty Menus

BREAKFAST	CALORIES
½ grapefruit	50
Oatmeal Granola*, with	155
½ cup skim milk	45
Decaf or herb tea	0

LUNCH	
Barley Bean Soup*	78
Eggplant Lasagna*	225
Lettuce and tomato salad	40
1 tablespoon Tomato Juice Salad Dressing*	3
1 slice whole grain bread	50
½ cup unsweetened fruit	100
Decaf or herb tea	0

MID-AFTERNOON SNACK	
1 fruit	100

DINNER	
Celery Pastina Soup*	89
Turkey Banana Loaf*	163
1 baked potato, with	90
2 tablespoons plain nonfat yogurt	30
½ cup cooked green beans	15
High C Salad*	46
Graham Carrot Muffin*	167
Decaf or herb tea	0

BEDTIME SNACK	
2 cups popped corn	100
½ cup fruit juice	50
Total	**1596**

PART II

RECIPES

—— 1 ——

Appetizers and Snacks

Crudites and Dip

2 carrots, scraped, cut into 3-inch sticks
½ pound green beans, washed, trimmed
1 cup broccoli flowerets
1 cup cauliflower flowerets
1 cup plain nonfat yogurt
½ teaspoon Worcestershire sauce
½ teaspoon prepared white horseradish
1 tablespoon grated Parmesan cheese

Arrange vegetables on a platter. Crisp in the refrigerator until ready to serve. For a dip, combine yogurt, Worcestershire sauce, horseradish, and grated Parmesan cheese. Place in center of vegetable platter.

SERVES: 8
CALORIES PER SERVING: 39

NUTRITION PER SERVING

Carbohydrate: .... 6 g	Cholesterol: .... 1 mg	Potassium: .... 230 mg
Protein: .... 3 g	Fiber: .... .8 g	Calcium: .... 129 mg
Total Fat: .... .2 g	Sodium: .... 18 mg	Iron: .... .5 mg

Chopped Eggplant

1 eggplant
1 sliced onion
1 green pepper, cut up
1 tablespoon olive oil
1 tablespoon fresh lemon juice
1 teaspoon red wine vinegar
¼ teaspoon thyme
¼ teaspoon pepper

Preheat oven to 350F. Bake the whole eggplant until the skin is soft and wrinkled. Remove from oven and cut skin away. Chop in a large chopping bowl. Add onion and green pepper and chop very fine. Add oil, lemon juice, thyme, and pepper. Mix well. Refrigerate. Serve in a mound on lettuce leaves.

SERVES: 8
CALORIES PER SERVING: 27

NUTRITION PER SERVING

Carbohydrate: .... 3 g	Cholesterol: .... 0 mg	Potassium: .... mg
Protein: .... 6 g	Fiber: .... .5 g	Calcium: .... 8 mg
Total Fat: .... 1.6 g	Sodium: .... mg	Iron: .... 2.8 mg

Spinach Stuffed Mushrooms

1 package (10 ounce) frozen chopped spinach, thawed
12 large mushrooms, 2-inch diameter
1 tablespoon chopped fresh parsley
⅛ teaspoon pepper
⅛ teaspoon ground nutmeg
¼ cup wheat germ

Drain thawed spinach in a strainer and press out all excess moisture. Wash mushrooms and carefully remove stems. Chop stems. Combine stems with parsley, pepper and nutmeg. Stuff mixture into mushroom caps. Place mushrooms, stuffing side up, in a small baking dish. Top each with a teaspoon of wheat germ. Bake for 15 minutes in a 350F. oven.

YIELD: 12 stuffed mushrooms
CALORIES PER SERVING: 17

NUTRITION PER SERVING

Carbohydrate: ....2 g	Cholesterol: .... 0 mg	Potassium: .... 143 mg
Protein:..............2 g	Fiber: ....3 g	Calcium:............ mg
Total Fat: ....5 g	Sodium: .... 13 mg	Iron: .... .8 mg

Oatmeal Granola

3 cups uncooked old-fashioned oats
1½ cups wheat germ
½ cup chopped almonds
½ cup sesame seeds
¼ cup hulled sunflower seeds
¼ cup honey

Combine all ingredients. Mix well. Spread mixture evenly in a nonstick baking pan. Bake in a 300 ° F oven for 30 minutes, stirring occasionally, until lightly toasted. Cool. Serve with skim milk as breakfast food, or use it for a snack.

YIELD: 6 cups
CALORIES PER ½ CUP SERVING: 155

NUTRITION PER SERVING

Carbohydrate: ....19 g	Cholesterol: .... none	Potassium: ....227 mg
Protein:..............7 g	Fiber: ....6 g	Calcium:..........28 mg
Total Fat: ....7 g	Sodium: ....132 mg	Iron: .... 1.9 mg

Munch Bowl

4 cups fresh air-popped corn
1 cup seedless raisins
2 cups puffed wheat cereal
½ cup hulled sunflower seeds
½ teaspoon ground cinnamon

Combine all ingredients and mix well.

YIELD: 15 Half-Cup Servings
CALORIES PER SERVING: 69

NUTRITION PER SERVING

Carbohydrate: .... 11 g	Cholesterol: .... none	Potassium: .... 125 mg
Protein: .... 2 g	Fiber: .... .3 g	Calcium: .... 13 mg
Total Fat: .... 2.3 g	Sodium: .... 4 mg	Iron: .... .8 mg

Tofu Banana Shake

1 pound tofu
1 cup water
3 ice cubes
1 banana
1 tablespoon honey
1 teaspoon vanilla extract

Combine all ingredients in a blender. Blend until smooth and creamy. Serve at once.

SERVES: 2

CALORIES PER SERVING: 247

NUTRITION PER SERVING

Carbohydrate: .... 26 g	Cholesterol: .... none	Potassium: .... 225 mg
Protein: .... 19 g	Fiber: .... .3 g	Calcium: .... 5 mg
Total Fat: .... 9 g	Sodium: .... 1 mg	Iron: .... 4.5 mg

—2—

Breakfast Dishes

Banana Pancakes

2 ripe bananas, mashed
½ cup uncooked oatmeal
½ cup unbleached flour
½ cup cornmeal
2 teaspoons baking powder
1½ cups skim milk
1 egg white, slightly beaten
1 teaspoon vanilla extract

Combine all ingredients and mix until well blended. Spoon ¼ cup of batter onto a preheated nonstick griddle. Repeat until griddle is filled with pancakes. Cook over medium heat. Brown on one side, turn and brown other side. Continue to make pancakes in this fashion until all batter is used. Serve with pureed fresh berries, if desired.

SERVES: 4
CALORIES PER SERVING: 120

NUTRITION PER SERVING

Carbohydrate: . . . . 16 g Cholesterol: . . . . . . 1.5 mg Potassium: . . . . 642 mg
Protein: . . . . 5 g Fiber: . . . . .4 g Calcium: . . . . 226 mg
Total Fat: . . . . .25 g Sodium: . . . . 159 mg Iron: . . . . .7 mg

Cottage Cheese Pancakes

²/₃ cup 1% low-fat cottage cheese
3 tablespoons flour
1 teaspoon vegetable oil
2 egg whites, beaten
¼ teaspoon cinnamon
½ teaspoon vanilla extract

Press cottage cheese through a strainer. Add flour and vegetable oil. Beat egg whites until soft peaks form; add to cheese mixture. Add cinnamon and vanilla extract. Drop by large spoonfuls onto a nonstick griddle or skillet. Cook over medium heat. When browned on one side, turn to brown the other side. Serve at once with unsweetened berries, if desired.

SERVES: 2

CALORIES PER SERVING: 131

NUTRITION PER SERVING

Carbohydrate:	10 g	Cholesterol:	3.5 mg	Potassium:	120 mg
Protein:	14 g	Fiber:	.05 g	Calcium:	52 mg
Total Fat:	2.5 g	Sodium:	48 mg	Iron:	4.5 mg

Cinnamon French Toast

1 egg white
½ cup skim milk
½ teaspoon vanilla extract
4 slices whole grain bread
Cinnamon

Beat egg white until frothy. Add skim milk and vanilla extract. Dip bread slices into the batter, one at a time, coating each side well. Place on a hot nonstick griddle or skillet surface. Cook over medium heat until browned on one side, then turn and brown other side. Lift to serving plates and sprinkle lightly with cinnamon.

SERVES: 4

CALORIES PER SERVING: 79

NUTRITION PER SERVING

Carbohydrate: ....15 g	Cholesterol: .... .5 mg	Potassium: ....134 mg
Protein:.............5 g	Fiber: ....4 g	Calcium:.........63 mg
Total Fat: ....1 g	Sodium: ....176 mg	Iron: ....8 mg

Oatmeal Raisin Pancakes

1 cup unbleached flour
½ cup uncooked oatmeal
1 tablespoon baking powder
1 cup skim milk
2 egg whites
1 tablespoon vegetable oil
1 teaspoon vanilla extract
¼ cup seedless raisins

Combine flour, oatmeal, and baking powder. Add milk, egg whites, oil, and vanilla extract. Add raisins. Stir until mixed through. Spoon ¼ cup of batter onto a hot nonstick griddle. Repeat until all batter is used. Cook on medium heat. Turn over when browned on underside. Serve at once with pureed berries as a topping, if desired. Makes 12 pancakes.

SERVES: 6

CALORIES PER SERVING: 145

NUTRITION PER SERVING

Carbohydrate: ....25 g	Cholesterol: .... .7 mg	Potassium: ....163 mg
Protein:.............5 g	Fiber: ....2 g	Calcium:.........90 mg
Total Fat: ....2.5 g	Sodium: ....247 mg	Iron: ....9 mg

Egg White Cottage Cheese Omelet

3 egg whites
¼ teaspoon dried dillweed
¼ cup 1% low-fat cottage cheese
½ teaspoon chopped chives
Dash pepper

Beat egg whites lightly with a fork until foamy. Add dillweed. Pour into a nonstick skillet. Cook over medium heat until whites are almost solidified.

179

Spoon cottage cheese over half the omelet, cover with other half. Roll out onto a plate. Sprinkle with chopped chives and a dusting of pepper.

SERVES: 1

CALORIES PER SERVING: 86

NUTRITION PER SERVING

Carbohydrate:	2 g	Cholesterol:	3 mg	Potassium:	183 mg
Protein:	16 g	Fiber:	none	Calcium:	47 mg
Total Fat:	1 g	Sodium:	144 mg	Iron:	.1 mg

Apricots and Grains

4 cups water
2 cups quick-cooking oatmeal
½ cup finely chopped dried apricots
1 teaspoon cinnamon
1 tablespoon frozen apple juice concentrate
½ cup wheat germ
Skim milk (optional)

Bring water to a boil in a large saucepan. Gradually stir in oatmeal, dried apricots, and cinnamon. Simmer, stirring occasionally, until oatmeal is thickened. Remove from heat. Stir in apple juice concentrate and wheat germ. Serve at once with skim milk, if desired.

SERVES: 4

CALORIES PER SERVING: 149 (no milk)

NUTRITION PER SERVING

Carbohydrate:	26 g	Cholesterol:	none	Potassium:	301 mg
Protein:	7 g	Fiber:	.8 g	Calcium:	25 mg
Total Fat:	3.2 g	Sodium:	132 mg	Iron:	1.2 mg

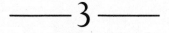

3

Soups

Barley Bean Soup

1 cup Great Northern dried beans
½ cup barley
1 onion, sliced thin
2 carrots, scraped and sliced
2 stalks celery, sliced
2 parsnips, scraped and sliced
1 turnip, peeled and cut into chunks
2 cloves garlic, minced
1 sprig dillweed
1 sprig parsley
1 teaspoon dried basil
½ teaspoon pepper

Soak beans for 1 hour. Pour off water. Add remaining ingredients and cover with 2 quarts water. Cover and cook over low heat for 3 hours, or until beans are tender. Stir occasionally.

SERVES: 10

CALORIES PER SERVING: 78

NUTRITION PER SERVING

Carbohydrate: ....17 g	Cholesterol: .... none	Potassium: ....261 mg
Protein:............ 2.7 g	Fiber: ....98 g	Calcium:.......... 35 mg
Total Fat: ....3 g	Sodium: ....26 mg	Iron: .... 1.1 mg

Black Bean Soup

1 pound dried black beans
2 quarts water
2 tablespoons olive oil
6 cloves garlic, diced
2 onions, diced
6 sweet chili peppers, seeded and chopped
¼ teaspoon pepper
¼ teaspoon dried oregano
¼ teaspoon ground cumin
2 bay leaves
1½ tablespoons vinegar
1 tablespoon frozen apple juice concentrate

Wash beans well, discarding any shriveled ones. Soak in water overnight. Drain beans, rinse in fresh water, and drain again. Place in a large heavy pot with 2 quarts water. Bring to a boil, then reduce heat, cover and cook 45 minutes. Heat oil in a nonstick skillet; sauté garlic, onions and chili peppers for 10 minutes, stirring occasionally. Add to skillet 1 drained cup of the cooked black beans and mash all together. Pour this mixture into cooked beans in pot. Add pepper, oregano, cumin, and bay leaves. Mix well, cover and cook over low heat for 1 hour. Add vinegar and apple juice concentrate. Serve with additional chopped onion on top, if desired.

SERVES: 8

CALORIES PER SERVING: 99

NUTRITION PER SERVING

Carbohydrate: .... 13 g	Cholesterol: .... none	Potassium: .... 251 mg
Protein: .... 4 g	Fiber: .... .8 g	Calcium: .... 31 mg
Total Fat: .... 3.5 g	Sodium: .... 6 mg	Iron: .... 1.4 mg

Cabbage Soup

4 beef bones, no meat
2 quarts water
2 sliced onions
1 medium cabbage, thinly sliced
4 large tomatoes, cut up
¼ cup white seedless raisins
¼ cup lemon juice
2 tablespoons frozen apple juice concentrate
½ teaspoon pepper
2 bay leaves

Place beef bones and water in a heavy pot. Add onions, cabbage, tomatoes, raisins, lemon juice, apple juice concentrate, pepper, and bay leaves. Bring to a boil, then reduce heat and simmer, covered, 2 to 3 hours.

SERVES: 8
CALORIES PER SERVING: 46

NUTRITION PER SERVING

Carbohydrate: .... 11 g	Cholesterol: .... none	Potassium: .... 310 mg
Protein: .... 1.3 g	Fiber: .... .8 g	Calcium: .... 33 mg
Total Fat: .... trace	Sodium: .... 12 mg	Iron: .... .7 mg

Celery Pastina Soup

2 cups diced celery
1 small onion, finely diced
1 potato, peeled and quartered
½ cup water
2 cups skim milk
¼ teaspoon marjoram
⅛ teaspoon pepper
¼ cup fine pastina

Simmer diced celery, onion, and potato in ½ cup water in small saucepan until vegetables are tender. Pour into a food processor and blend until smooth. Add 1 cup skim milk and blend again. Pour into a saucepan; add remaining milk, marjoram, pepper, and pastina. Simmer and stir until hot and thickened.

SERVES: 4

CALORIES PER SERVING: 89

NUTRITION PER SERVING

Carbohydrate: .... 16 g	Cholesterol: .... 2 mg	Potassium: .... 526 mg
Protein: .... 6 g	Fiber: .... .6 g	Calcium: .... 180 mg
Total Fat: .... trace	Sodium: .... 141 mg	Iron: .... .5 mg

Salt-Free Chicken Broth

1 chicken, about 3 pounds
2 quarts water
1 large onion, peeled
4 carrots, scraped
2 stalks celery with leaves
2 parsnips, scraped
1 sprig parsley
1 sprig dillweed
¼ teaspoon ground white pepper
¼ teaspoon thyme
1 bay leaf

Wash and clean chicken; place in a heavy pot with lid. Add water, onion, carrots, celery, parsnips, parsley, dillweed, pepper, thyme, and bay leaf. Simmer 1½ hours. Remove chicken. Strain broth through a fine sieve. Discard celery, parsley, dillweed, and onion. Slice carrots and parsnips and return to the soup. Remove chicken from bones and add to soup. Chill soup to allow fat to solidify on top, then remove fat and discard before reheating soup.

SERVES: 8
CALORIES PER SERVING: 155 (with vegetables and chicken)

NUTRITION PER SERVING

Carbohydrate: ....21 g	Cholesterol: .... 66 mg	Potassium: .... 592 mg
Protein:.............14 g	Fiber: .... 1.8 g	Calcium:.......... 74 mg
Total Fat: .... 1.8 g	Sodium: .... 66 mg	Iron: .... 2 mg

Cream of Cucumber Soup

2 cucumbers, peeled
1 cup salt-free chicken broth (see p. 185)
½ cup nonfat plain yogurt
½ cup skim milk
½ cup buttermilk
1 scallion, thinly sliced, including tops
1 tablespoon chopped fresh parsley
¼ teaspoon dried dillweed
⅛ teaspoon Tabasco sauce

Cut cucumbers lengthwise and remove seeds. Place all ingredients in an electric food processor or blender; process until pureed. Chill until ready to serve.

SERVES: 6

CALORIES PER SERVING: 30

NUTRITION PER SERVING

Carbohydrate: .... 4 g	Cholesterol: ...... 1.5 mg	Potassium: .... 149 mg
Protein: .... 2.5 g	Fiber: .... .3 g	Calcium: .... 93 mg
Total Fat: .... .2 g	Sodium: .... 39 mg	Iron: .... .3 mg

Fish Chowder

2 peeled and cubed potatoes
1 onion, thinly sliced
1 sprig dillweed, finely chopped
2 cups water
1 pound fish fillets, such as flounder or cod
2 cups skim milk
¼ teaspoon dried thyme
¼ teaspoon white pepper

Simmer potatoes, onions, and dillweed in water, covered in large saucepan, until potatoes are soft, about 15 minutes. Cut fish fillets into small chunks and add to the potatoes. Stir in milk, thyme, and pepper. Simmer, covered, for an additional 15–20 minutes, stirring occasionally. Serve at once.

SERVES: 8

CALORIES PER SERVING: 163

NUTRITION PER SERVING

Carbohydrate: .... 14 g	Cholesterol: .... 34 mg	Potassium: .... 435 mg
Protein:............. 19 g	Fiber: .... .3 g	Calcium:......... 107 mg
Total Fat: .... 3.2 g	Sodium: .... 99 mg	Iron: .... .9 mg

Gazpacho

4 large tomatoes, cut up
1 clove garlic, peeled
1 cucumber, peeled, cut up
1 green pepper, seeded, cut up
2 scallions with tops, sliced
2 tablespoons wine vinegar
1 egg white
1 tablespoon frozen concentrated apple juice
¼ teaspoon pepper

Place all ingredients into an electric food processor or blender. Process, but do not puree completely. Chill. Serve with additional diced cucumber and sliced scallions on top, if desired.

SERVES: 4

CALORIES PER SERVING: 43

NUTRITION PER SERVING

Carbohydrate: .... 10 g	Cholesterol: .... none	Potassium: .... 402 mg
Protein: .... 2 g	Fiber: .... 4.3 g	Calcium: .... 25 mg
Total Fat: .... trace	Sodium: .... 20 mg	Iron: .... 1 mg

Lima Barley Soup

1 cup dried small lima beans
½ cup barley
2 cups chopped tomatoes
4 carrots, scraped and sliced
4 stalks celery, thinly sliced
2 onions, thinly sliced
1 clove garlic, finely minced
1 bay leaf
2 whole cloves
1 tablespoon lemon juice
¼ teaspoon pepper

In a heavy soup pot, soak beans covered with water for several hours or overnight. Drain. Add remaining ingredients and 2 quarts fresh water. Bring to a boil, reduce heat, cover and simmer 3 hours, or until beans are tender.

SERVES: 10
CALORIES PER SERVING: 102

NUTRITION PER SERVING

Carbohydrate: .... 21 g	Cholesterol: .... none	Potassium: .... 451 mg
Protein: .... 5 g	Fiber: .... 1.3 g	Calcium: .... 30 mg
Total Fat: .... .4 g	Sodium: .... 27 mg	Iron: .... 1.7 mg

Curried Split Pea Soup

2 cups dried split peas
2½ quarts water
1 large carrot, grated
2 medium potatoes, grated
1 large onion, grated
1 teaspoon curry powder
¼ teaspoon pepper

Wash split peas, drain, and place in a large kettle with a tight-fitting lid. Add water, carrot, potatoes, onion, curry powder, and pepper. Cover and bring to a boil; then lower heat and simmer for about 2 hours, or until peas are soft. Stir until peas fall apart, or press soup through a strainer.

SERVES: 10
CALORIES PER SERVING: 62

NUTRITION PER SERVING

Carbohydrate: .... 12 g	Cholesterol: .... none	Potassium: .... 229 mg
Protein:............. 3 g	Fiber: .... .8 g	Calcium:.......... 15 mg
Total Fat: .... .2 g	Sodium: .... 9 mg	Iron: .... .9 mg

Potato Soup

1 pound potatoes
1 medium onion
1 quart water
¹/₂ cup skim milk
1 cup nonfat yogurt
¹/₈ teaspoon pepper
1 tablespoon chopped fresh parsley
¹/₂ teaspoon paprika

Peel and slice the potatoes and onion. Put into a saucepan with water; cover
and bring to a boil. Reduce heat and simmer until vegetables are soft, about
35 minutes. Pour water and vegetables into an electric blender and blend at
high speed. Stir in milk, yogurt, and pepper. Heat on low temperature, but
do not boil. Serve with a sprinkling of chopped parsley and paprika.

SERVES: 8
CALORIES PER SERVING: 60

NUTRITION PER SERVING

Carbohydrate: .... 12 g	Cholesterol: .... .7 mg	Potassium: .... 268 mg
Protein: .... 3 g	Fiber: .... .4 g	Calcium: .... 83 mg
Total Fat: .... trace	Sodium: .... 11 mg	Iron: .... .4 mg

Tomato Rice Soup

8 large fresh tomatoes
3 beef marrow bones, no meat
2 quarts water
2 onions, finely diced
1 clove garlic, finely minced
½ teaspoon paprika
¼ teaspoon pepper
¼ teaspoon dried basil
2 tablespoons lemon juice
1 tablespoon cider vinegar
2 tablespoons frozen apple juice concentrate
3 tablespoons cream of rice cereal
½ cup uncooked rice

Briefly dip tomatoes into boiling water and peel them. Cut up and place in a deep pot. Add bones, water, onions, garlic, paprika, pepper, basil, lemon juice, vinegar, and apple juice concentrate. Simmer for 2 hours, covered. Stir some of the hot soup into the cream of rice cereal until smooth, then add this mixture to the soup, stirring as it thickens. Add rice and cook for 30 minutes more.

SERVES: 8

CALORIES PER SERVING: 96

NUTRITION PER SERVING

Carbohydrate: ..... 22.7 g	Cholesterol: .... none	Potassium: .... 352 mg
Protein: .... 2 g	Fiber: .... .87 g	Calcium: .... 26.7 mg
Total Fat: .... .125 g	Sodium: .... 18 mg	Iron: .... 1.3 mg

Vegetable Soup

1 large yellow turnip, peeled and diced
4 carrots, scraped and sliced
4 stalks celery, sliced
2 large onions, sliced
3 tomatoes, peeled and diced
1 garlic clove, minced
½ pound green beans, trimmed and cut up
2 quarts water
2 bay leaves
1 tablespoon wine vinegar
½ teaspoon pepper
½ teaspoon dried oregano

Place all ingredients in a large soup pot. Bring to a boil, then reduce heat and simmer, covered, for 2 hours.

SERVES: 12

CALORIES PER SERVING: 26

NUTRITION PER SERVING

Carbohydrate:	6 g	Cholesterol:	none	Potassium:	238 mg
Protein:	1 g	Fiber:	7 g	Calcium:	24 mg
Total Fat:	trace	Sodium:	57 mg	Iron:	.6 mg

—4—

Seafood Entrées

Herb Stuffed Sole

6 fillets of sole, about 1½ pounds
2 teaspoons prepared mustard
1 onion, finely diced
¾ cup wheat germ
¼ cup chopped fresh parsley
½ teaspoon dried thyme
½ teaspoon dried rosemary
⅛ teaspoon pepper

Place fillets of sole flat. Cover surface with a thin coating of mustard. Combine remaining ingredients and sprinkle over mustard. Roll up, jelly-roll fashion. Place in a nonstick baking pan. Bake in a 350° F oven for 25 minutes, or until cooked through.

SERVES: 6
CALORIES PER SERVING: 286

NUTRITION PER SERVING

Carbohydrate: ....7 g	Cholesterol: ....52 mg	Potassium: ....821 mg
Protein:............38 g	Fiber: ....4 g	Calcium:..........42 mg
Total Fat:...........11 g	Sodium: ....293 mg	Iron: ....2.8 mg

Sole Rolls with Vegetable Sauce

4 fillets of sole, about 1 pound
¼ cup lime juice
1 tablespoon chopped chives
1 tablespoon grated Parmesan cheese
2 tomatoes, chopped
1 zucchini, thinly sliced
1 green pepper, finely diced
1 onion, finely diced
½ teaspoon oregano
⅛ teaspoon white pepper
¼ cup white wine or water

Lay fillets of sole flat. Sprinkle with lime juice, chopped chives, and grated Parmesan cheese; roll up and set aside. In a large skillet, simmer tomatoes, zucchini, green pepper, onion, oregano, pepper, and wine for 3 minutes. Place prepared sole rolls in this mixture. Cover and cook over low heat for 5–7 minutes, or until fish flakes easily. Serve at once.

SERVES: 4
CALORIES PER SERVING: 268

NUTRITION PER SERVING

Carbohydrate: ....8 g	Cholesterol: ..... 53.2 mg	Potassium: .... 964 mg
Protein:.............36 g	Fiber: ....1 g	Calcium:.......... 76 mg
Total Fat: .... 9.7 g	Sodium: ....287 mg	Iron: .... 2.4 mg

Broiled Flounder Parmesan

1 pound fillets of flounder
2 tomatoes, skinned, chopped
1 tablespoon grated onion
¼ teaspoon dried oregano
⅛ teaspoon pepper
1 tablespoon grated Parmesan cheese

Arrange flounder fillets on a broiling pan. Spoon chopped tomatoes over the fish. Add grated onion, oregano, and pepper. Top with a sprinkling of Parmesan cheese. Broil 5–7 minutes, or until fish flakes easily.

SERVES: 4
CALORIES PER SERVING: 249

NUTRITION PER SERVING

Carbohydrate: ....3 g	Cholesterol: .... 53 mg	Potassium: .... 821 mg
Protein:.............35 g	Fiber: ....4 g	Calcium:.......... 56 mg
Total Fat: .... 9.7 g	Sodium: .... 282 mg	Iron: .... 1.9 mg

Flounder Creole

2 cups chopped tomatoes
1 can (8 ounce) tomato sauce
1 onion, finely diced
1 green pepper, finely diced
1 bay leaf
½ teaspoon thyme
⅛ teaspoon pepper
1 pound flounder fillets

Combine tomatoes, tomato sauce, onion, and green pepper in a saucepan. Add bay leaf, thyme, and pepper. Cook over low heat 15 minutes, stirring occasionally. Remove bay leaf. Arrange flounder fillets in a flat baking dish. Spoon sauce over fish. Bake at 375° F for 20 minutes, or until fish flakes easily.

SERVES: 4
CALORIES PER SERVING: 225

NUTRITION PER SERVING

Carbohydrate: .... 7 g	Cholesterol: .... 52 mg	Potassium: .... 779 mg
Protein: .... 34 g	Fiber: .... .8 g	Calcium: .... 47 mg
Total Fat: .... 6 g	Sodium: .... 285 mg	Iron: .... 2 mg

Flounder with Broccoli Stuffing

1 small stalk broccoli
1 carrot, grated
⅛ teaspoon ground nutmeg
⅛ teaspoon pepper
2 slices fillet of flounder, about ½ pound
1 tablespoon lemon juice
¼ cup dry white wine
¼ teaspoon paprika

Cut up broccoli and simmer in a small amount of water for several minutes until tender. Drain. Chop broccoli fine and add grated carrot, nutmeg, and pepper. Spread mixture over the top of each piece of fish and roll up. Place in a small skillet or saucepan. Add lemon juice and white wine. Dust top of fish rolls with paprika. Cover and cook over medium heat for 5–7 minutes, or until fish flakes easily. Remove stuffed fish rolls to a platter.

SERVES: 2

CALORIES PER SERVING: 268

NUTRITION PER SERVING

Carbohydrate: .:...... 8 g	Cholesterol: .... 52 mg	Potassium: .... 444 mg
Protein: .... 37 g	Fiber: .... 1.7 g	Calcium: .... 119 mg
Total Fat: .... 10 g	Sodium: .... 295 mg	Iron: .... 2.5 mg

Broiled Lemon Flounder and Tomato

4 slices fillet of flounder, about 1 pound
1 lemon
½ teaspoon dried dillweed
¼ teaspoon paprika
2 tomatoes, cut in half through diameter
1 tablespoon chopped fresh parsley
2 tablespoons whole grain bread crumbs
1 teaspoon grated Parmesan cheese

Place fish in a nonstick baking pan. Squeeze lemon juice over fish. Sprinkle with dillweed and paprika. Place halves of tomatoes, cut side up, in the baking dish next to the fish. Top tomato halves with parsley, bread crumbs, and a sprinkling of grated Parmesan cheese. Broil 7–8 minutes, or until fish flakes easily.

SERVES: 4
CALORIES PER SERVING: 260

NUTRITION PER SERVING

Carbohydrate: .... 7 g	Cholesterol: ..... 52.5 mg	Potassium: .... 853 mg
Protein:............. 35 g	Fiber: .... .4 g	Calcium:.......... 51 mg
Total Fat: .... 9.7 g	Sodium: .... 298 mg	Iron: .... 2.1 mg

Baked Cod Oreganata

1 pound cod fillets
1 tablespoon olive oil
1 clove garlic, finely minced
1 small onion, finely diced
½ green pepper, finely diced
3 tomatoes, chopped
½ teaspoon oregano
⅛ teaspoon pepper
½ cup dry white wine

Arrange cod fillets in one layer in a flat baking dish. Combine olive oil, garlic, onion, green pepper, tomatoes, oregano, and pepper. Spread mixture lightly over cod fish. Pour wine around fish. Bake, uncovered, in a 350° F oven for 25–30 minutes, or until fish flakes easily.

SERVES: 4

CALORIES PER SERVING: 248

NUTRITION PER SERVING

Carbohydrate: .... 6 g	Cholesterol: .... 66 mg	Potassium: .... 727 mg
Protein: .... 33 g	Fiber: .... .7 g	Calcium: .... 51 mg
Total Fat: .... 9 g	Sodium: .... 130 mg	Iron: .... 1.7 mg

Halibut Mousse

1 cup skim milk
2 cups bread crumbs
1 pound raw halibut, ground or chopped fine
½ teaspoon nutmeg
¼ teaspoon white pepper
4 egg whites

Preheat oven to 350° F. Stir milk into bread crumbs. Add ground fish, nutmeg and pepper. Beat egg whites separately until stiff; fold into fish mixture. Spoon mixture into a nonstick 8½ × 4½–inch loaf pan. Place this pan in a larger pan with one inch of hot water. Bake 45 minutes, or until firm. Let stand 10 minutes before slicing.

SERVES: 8

CALORIES PER SERVING: 230

NUTRITION PER SERVING

Carbohydrate:	20 g	Cholesterol:	52.5 mg	Potassium:	444 mg
Protein:	23 g	Fiber:	.07 g	Calcium:	83 mg
Total Fat:	5.9 g	Sodium:	358 mg	Iron:	1.7 mg

Stuffed Baked Red Snapper

1 whole red snapper, about 4 pounds, cleaned
2 tablespoons margarine
1 small onion, diced
1 cup dry bread, torn up
1 apple, peeled and diced
½ cup seedless white raisins
2 tablespoons chopped fresh parsley
¼ cup skim milk
1 egg white
¼ teaspoon thyme
⅛ teaspoon pepper
Juice of 1 lemon

Wash and wipe fish dry. In a saucepan, melt margarine and sauté diced onion until golden and translucent. Add the bread, diced apple, raisins, and parsley. Combine milk and egg white; add to bread mixture. Add thyme and pepper. Stir lightly so mixture does not pack down. Fill cavity of fish with this mixture. Place fish in a nonstick baking dish. Squeeze lemon juice over the fish. Bake in a 350° F oven for 45 minutes, or until fish flakes easily.

SERVES: 6
CALORIES PER SERVING: 268

NUTRITION PER SERVING

Carbohydrate: ....19 g	Cholesterol: .... 52 mg	Potassium: .... 636 mg
Protein:.............25 g	Fiber: .... .5 g	Calcium:.......... 54 mg
Total Fat: ....10 g	Sodium: .... 287 mg	Iron: .... 1.9 mg

Poached Salmon Veronique

2 thin center slices fresh salmon
1 cup water
¼ cup cider vinegar
1 onion, sliced thin
1 sprig dillweed
3 whole cloves
1 bay leaf
1 peppercorn
½ cup seedless green grapes
2 lemon wedges

Place salmon slices in a large skillet. Add water, vinegar, onion, dillweed, cloves, bay leaf, and peppercorn. Bring to a boil, then reduce heat and simmer, covered, 6–10 minutes, or until salmon is cooked through. Add grapes, cover and cook 1 minute more. Remove with a slotted spatula. Serve garnished with the grapes, lemon wedges, and additional sprigs of dill.

SERVES: 2

CALORIES PER SERVING: 225

NUTRITION PER SERVING

Carbohydrate: . . . . . . .15 g	Cholesterol: . . . . 52 mg	Potassium: . . . . 584 mg
Protein:. . . . . .24 g	Fiber: . . . . .5 g	Calcium:. . . . . 241 mg
Total Fat: . . . . 7 g	Sodium: . . . . 444 mg	Iron: . . . . 1.6 mg

Monkfish in Mushroom Cream Sauce

1 pound boneless monkfish
1 green pepper, seeded, thinly sliced
½ cup sliced mushrooms
2 tablespoons chopped chives
1 tablespoon chopped fresh parsley
½ cup white wine or water
1 lemon
¼ cup evaporated skim milk
1 tablespoon cornstarch
¼ teaspoon paprika

Cut monkfish into 1–inch thick slices. Place fish in a large nonstick skillet. Add diced green pepper, sliced mushrooms, chives, parsley, wine, and the juice of 1 lemon. Cover and cook over low heat 5–7 minutes, or until cooked through. Remove fish to a hot platter. Combine evaporated skim milk and cornstarch; mix until smooth. Stir into fish liquid. Cook and stir until liquid is thickened. Pour over fish. Sprinkle with paprika. Serve at once.

SERVES: 4

CALORIES PER SERVING: 243

NUTRITION PER SERVING

Carbohydrate: . . . . .7 g	Cholesterol: . . . . 67 mg	Potassium: . . . . 643 mg
Protein:. . . . . .34 g	Fiber: . . . . .4 g	Calcium:. . . . . 84 mg
Total Fat: . . . . 6 g	Sodium: . . . . 147 mg	Iron: . . . . 1.6 mg

Sautéed Oysters

1 pint fresh shelled oysters with juice
2 tablespoons finely chopped celery
2 tablespoons finely chopped green pepper
1 tablespoon finely chopped fresh parsley
2 teaspoons lemon juice
¼ teaspoon ground thyme
⅛ teaspoon ground white pepper

Pour oysters and juice into a large nonstick skillet. Add celery, green pepper, parsley, lemon juice, thyme, and pepper. Cook over low heat and stir until edges of oysters begin to curl, about 3 minutes. Serve over toast points, if desired.

SERVES: 4
CALORIES PER SERVING: 82

NUTRITION PER SERVING

Carbohydrate: .... 5 g	Cholesterol: .... 60 mg	Potassium: .... 177 mg
Protein: .... 10 g	Fiber: .... .1 g	Calcium: .... 117 mg
Total Fat: .... 2 g	Sodium: .... 93 mg	Iron: .... 6.7 mg

Linguine with Scallops

8 ounces linguine
1 tablespoon olive oil
1 clove garlic, finely minced
1 cup clam juice
1 can (28 ounce) Italian plum tomatoes
½ teaspoon dried thyme
1 pound bay or sea scallops

Cook linguine as directed on package. Drain. Meanwhile, heat oil in a nonstick skillet; sauté garlic until golden. Add clam juice. Chop tomatoes and add to skillet. Add thyme. About 3 minutes before the pasta is done, add the scallops to the sauce. (If using sea scallops, cut into small pieces.) Cook scallops about 3 minutes, or until they are opaque. Place drained pasta on a heated serving dish; spoon scallops and sauce over pasta.

SERVES: 4

CALORIES PER SERVING: 384

NUTRITION PER SERVING

Carbohydrate: . . . . 48 g	Cholesterol: . . . . 52 mg	Potassium: . . . . . . 1097 mg
Protein: . . . . 4 g	Fiber: . . . . 1.1 g	Calcium: . . . . 169 mg
Total Fat: . . . . 5.7 g	Sodium: . . . . 308 mg	Iron: . . . . 5.7 mg

Scallops Cacciatore on Pasta

1 pound scallops
1 onion, diced
1 green pepper, diced
1 clove garlic, minced
1 can (16 ounce) unsalted tomatoes
1 bay leaf
1 tablespoon chopped parsley
⅛ teaspoon pepper
8 ounces spaghetti
3 quarts boiling water

Rinse scallops in cold water and remove any clinging bits of shell. Place in a nonstick skillet with onion, green pepper, garlic, tomatoes, bay leaf, parsley, and pepper. Cook over low heat for 5 minutes, or until scallops are cooked through. Meanwhile, cook spaghetti in boiling water 9–12 minutes, until tender; drain. Add spaghetti to the skillet, mix through, and serve at once.

SERVES: 4

CALORIES PER SERVING: 312

NUTRITION PER SERVING

Carbohydrate: . . . . 39 g	Cholesterol: . . . . 52 mg	Potassium: . . . . 952 mg
Protein: . . . . 65 g	Fiber: . . . . .9 g	Calcium: . . . . 162 mg
Total Fat: 5g	Sodium: . . . . 307 mg	Iron: . . . . 5.4 mg

Linguine with White Clam Sauce

1 tablespoon olive oil
2 cloves garlic, finely minced
³/₄ cup clam juice
¹/₄ cup dry white wine
2 tablespoons chopped parsley
¹/₂ teaspoon oregano
¹/₄ teaspoon pepper
1¹/₂ cups minced cooked clams
8 ounces linguine, cooked, drained
2 tablespoons grated Parmesan cheese

Heat oil in a large nonstick skillet over medium heat. Add garlic, stirring frequently; cook 1 minute. Add clam juice, wine, parsley, oregano, and pepper. Stirring occasionally, simmer 10 minutes. Stir in clams; cook 3 minutes longer. Place cooked linguine on a hot platter, top with clam sauce and then sprinkle with grated Parmesan cheese. Serve at once.

SERVES: 4
CALORIES PER SERVING: 300

NUTRITION PER SERVING

Carbohydrate: ....41 g	Cholesterol: .... 44 mg	Potassium: ....281 mg
Protein:.............19 g	Fiber: ....1 g	Calcium:.........119 mg
Total Fat: .... 6.2 g	Sodium: .... 127 mg	Iron: .... 6.7 mg

—5—
Poultry Entrées

Chicken Paprikash

1 broiler chicken, cut into parts
2 teaspoons sweet paprika
1 tablespoon olive oil
1 onion, thinly sliced
1 clove garlic, finely minced
1 cup salt-free chicken broth (see page 185)
2 teaspoons cornstarch
2 tablespoons water

Wash the chicken parts and pat dry. Sprinkle with paprika on all sides. Heat oil in a large nonstick skillet; sauté onion and garlic until limp. Push onion aside and sear chicken parts on all sides, continuously turning the pieces as you cook over medium heat. Add broth. Cover and cook over low heat for 1 hour. Combine cornstarch and water into a thin paste. Spoon some of the hot gravy into the paste, stir until smooth, then return to the skillet, stirring continuously. Cook and stir until gravy is thickened and transparent. Do not eat skin.

SERVES: 4
CALORIES PER SERVING: 163

NUTRITION PER SERVING

Carbohydrate: . . . . .3 g	Cholesterol: . . . . . . 131 mg	Potassium: . . . . . . .279 mg
Protein:. . . . . .21 g	Fiber: . . . . .1 g	Calcium:. . . . . 14 mg
Total Fat: . . . . 6.7 g	Sodium: . . . . 60 mg	Iron: . . . . 1.6 mg

Baked Chicken and Pineapple

4 chicken breast halves, skin removed
1 can (13½ ounce) unsweetened pineapple chunks in juice
½ cup whole-wheat bread crumbs
2 tablespoons chopped fresh parsley
¼ teaspoon ground ginger
¼ teaspoon nutmeg

Dip chicken breasts in pineapple juice. Combine bread crumbs, parsley, ginger, and nutmeg. Coat chicken with this mixture. Place in a flat nonstick baking pan. Spoon pineapple chunks around chicken pieces and pour remaining juice over all. Bake in a 350° F oven for 1 hour.

SERVES: 4

CALORIES PER SERVING: 290

NUTRITION PER SERVING

Carbohydrate: . . . . . . .20 g	Cholesterol: . . . . 60 mg	Potassium: . . . . . . .472 mg
Protein:. . . . . .38 g	Fiber: . . . . .6 g	Calcium:. . . . . 42 mg
Total Fat: . . . . .6 g	Sodium: . . . . 148 mg	Iron: . . . . 2.3 mg

Poached Chicken Florentine

4 boneless, skinless chicken breast halves, about 1 pound
1 cup water
1 tablespoon fresh lemon juice
1 sprig fresh dillweed
1 small onion, thinly sliced
1 carrot, scraped and grated
1 pound fresh spinach, washed, trimmed
½ teaspoon nutmeg
⅛ teaspoon pepper

Arrange chicken breast halves in a large skillet. Pour water around chicken. Add lemon juice, dillweed, onion, and carrot. Cover and simmer gently for 20 minutes, or until chicken is cooked through. Remove chicken to a heated plate and reserve. Place washed spinach with clinging water, nutmeg, and pepper into same skillet containing chicken cooking liquid. Cover and cook for several minutes, just until the spinach is limp. Place poached chicken over the spinach and rewarm for a minute or two. Serve chicken over a bed of cooked spinach.

SERVES: 4

CALORIES PER SERVING: 228

NUTRITION PER SERVING

Carbohydrate: .... 6 g	Cholesterol: .... 60 mg	Potassium: .... 577 mg
Protein:............ 38 g	Fiber: .... .4 g	Calcium:.......... 50 mg
Total Fat: .... 5.2 g	Sodium: .... 85 mg	Iron: .... 2.6 mg

Chicken Mexicana

¾ cup uncooked brown rice
1 tablespoon olive oil
1 tomato, peeled and diced
1 onion, finely diced
1 clove garlic, finely diced
1 broiler chicken, cut up, about 2½ pounds
2 cups water
½ teaspoon chili powder
¼ teaspoon pepper

In a nonstick skillet, brown rice in olive oil, stirring constantly. Add tomatoes, onion, and garlic. Cook and stir for several minutes. Place chicken parts in a heavy saucepan. Add rice mixture, water, chili powder, and pepper. Bring to a boil. Lower heat, cover and simmer about 25 minutes, until chicken and rice are tender.

SERVES: 4

CALORIES PER SERVING: 287

NUTRITION PER SERVING

Carbohydrate: .... 30 g	Cholesterol: ...... 131 mg	Potassium: .... 417 mg
Protein:............ 24 g	Fiber: .... 1.1 g	Calcium:.......... 27 mg
Total Fat: .... 7 g	Sodium: .... 64 mg	Iron: .... 2.3 mg

Oven-Fried Lemon Chicken

8 broiler chicken thighs, skinned
½ cup nonfat lemon yogurt
½ teaspoon ground ginger
½ teaspoon garlic powder
½ cup whole-wheat bread crumbs

Dip each thigh into a mixture of yogurt, ginger, and garlic powder; then coat lightly with bread crumbs. Place in a single layer in a nonstick baking pan. Bake in a 350° F oven for 35 minutes, or until chicken is tender and coating is crisp.

SERVES: 4

CALORIES PER SERVING: 278

NUTRITION PER SERVING

Carbohydrate: .... 13 g	Cholesterol: .... 62 mg	Potassium: .... 85 mg
Protein: .... 29 g	Fiber: .... .05 g	Calcium: .... 79 mg
Total Fat: .... 11 g	Sodium: .... 106 mg	Iron: .... 2.5 mg

Chicken Stew

1 broiler chicken, cut into parts
2 cups chopped tomatoes
4 large potatoes, peeled, cut into chunks
8 small white onions, peeled
4 carrots, scraped, cut into chunks
1 large green pepper, seeded, diced
2 stalks celery, cut into chunks
2 sprigs parsley
1 bay leaf
½ teaspoon dried thyme
1 cup water
2 tablespoons cornstarch

Place chicken pieces in a large pot. Add tomatoes, potatoes, onions, carrots, green pepper, celery, parsley, bay leaf, thyme, and water. Simmer, covered, for 1 hour, or until chicken is tender. Stir cornstarch with just enough water to make a thin paste; spoon some of the hot liquid into the cornstarch, stir well and then return all to the pot. Stir constantly over medium heat until gravy thickens. Remove chicken skin before serving.

SERVES: 4
CALORIES PER SERVING: 285

NUTRITION PER SERVING

Carbohydrate: .... 38 g	Cholesterol: ...... 131 mg	Potassium: ..... 1,292 mg
Protein: .... 26 g	Fiber: .... 2.5 g	Calcium: .... 72 mg
Total Fat: .... 3.5 g	Sodium: .... 127 mg	Iron: .... 3.6 mg

Chicken Stroganoff

4 boneless, skinless chicken breast halves
¼ cup lemon juice
½ teaspoon paprika
½ cup water
1 sprig fresh parsley
¼ cup plain nonfat yogurt

Sprinkle chicken with lemon juice. Arrange chicken in a nonstick skillet. Sprinkle with paprika. Add water and parsley. Cover and simmer for 15 minutes, or until cooked through. Remove chicken to a warm platter. Stir yogurt into the cooking broth, then cook and stir over low heat to prevent curdling. Pour over chicken and serve.

SERVES: 4
CALORIES PER SERVING: 215

NUTRITION PER SERVING

Carbohydrate: .... 3 g	Cholesterol: .... 60 mg	Potassium: .... 411 mg
Protein: .... 37 g	Fiber: .... .05 g	Calcium: .... 43 mg
Total Fat: .... 5.2 g	Sodium: .... 55 mg	Iron: .... 1.6 mg

Sesame Chicken Kabobs

1 pound boned and skinned chicken breasts
¾ cup orange juice
1 tablespoon sesame seeds
1 tablespoon brown sugar
2 teaspoons grated orange peel
1 teaspoon ground ginger
½ teaspoon garlic powder
½ teaspoon onion powder
⅛ teaspoon ground red pepper
4 ounces fresh mushrooms, halved
1 green pepper, cut into 1-inch pieces

Pierce chicken with fork tines; cut into 1-inch pieces. In a small bowl, combine orange juice, sesame seeds, brown sugar, orange peel, ginger, garlic and onion powders, and red pepper. Add chicken, toss to coat and then marinate for 30 minutes. Preheat broiler to hot. Arrange chicken pieces on four 10-inch skewers, alternating with mushrooms and green peppers. Broil on a rack in a pan 3 to 4 inches from heat, until chicken is just cooked through, about 8 minutes. Brush frequently with marinade and turn chicken after 4 minutes.

SERVES: 4

CALORIES PER SERVING: 261

NUTRITION PER SERVING

Carbohydrate: 12	Cholesterol: .... 60 mg	Potassium: .... 608 mg
Protein:..............38 g	Fiber: .... 2.2 g	Calcium:.......... 26 mg
Total Fat: .... 5.2 g	Sodium: .... 63 mg	Iron: .... 2 mg

Roast Chicken with Prune Orange Stuffing

1 roaster chicken, about 4¹/₂ pounds
1 teaspoon dried thyme
¹/₂ teaspoon garlic powder
2 oranges
8 large pitted prunes
1 egg white
1¹/₂ cups dried bread cubes

Rub chicken with thyme and garlic powder, inside and outside. Chop the pulp of the oranges and the prunes; add the egg white and bread cubes. Mix well. If too dry, add a small amount of cool water or orange juice to the mixture. Stuff the mixture into the cavity of the chicken. Close opening with skewers. Roast on a rack in a roasting pan at 350° F for 2 hours, or until tender. Baste occasionally with pan drippings.

SERVES: 8

CALORIES PER SERVING: 178

NUTRITION PER SERVING

Carbohydrate: ....14 g	Cholesterol: ......131 mg	Potassium: ....391 mg
Protein:.............22 g	Fiber: .... .4 g	Calcium:.......... 32 mg
Total Fat: .... 3.7 g	Sodium: ....98 mg	Iron: .... 2.1 mg

Herb-Broiled Cornish Hens

2 Cornish hens, about 1 pound each
1 tablespoon olive oil
2 tablespoons lemon juice
1/8 teaspoon rosemary
1/8 teaspoon thyme
1/8 teaspoon pepper

Split hens in half. Place cut-side down on a broiling pan. Combine oil, lemon juice, rosemary, thyme, and pepper. Brush half of this mixture on top of hens and broil for 8 minutes. Turn hens and brush with remaining mixture. Broil for 8 minutes more, or until done. Remove skin before eating.

SERVES: 4
CALORIES PER SERVING: 151

NUTRITION PER SERVING

Carbohydrate: .... .5 g	Cholesterol: ...... 131 mg	Potassium: .... 252 mg
Protein: .... 21 g	Fiber: .... trace	Calcium: .... 8 mg
Total Fat: .... 6.7 g	Sodium: .... 58 mg	Iron: .... 1.5 mg

Broiled Turkey Cutlets Rosemary

4 turkey cutlets, about 1 pound
½ cup apricot nectar
½ teaspoon dried rosemary
¼ teaspoon ginger
⅛ teaspoon pepper

Arrange turkey cutlets on a broiling rack. Combine apricot nectar, rosemary, ginger, and pepper. Spoon half of the mixture over the cutlets. Broil 4 minutes. Turn cutlets and spoon remaining mixture over them. Broil 4 minutes more, or until done to your taste.

SERVES: 4
CALORIES PER SERVING: 213

NUTRITION PER SERVING

Carbohydrate: ...... 3.5 g	Cholesterol: .... 31 mg	Potassium: .... 541 mg
Protein: .... 37 g	Fiber: .... .1 g	Calcium: .... 4 mg
Total Fat: .... 4.2 g	Sodium: .... 93 mg	Iron: .... 1.5 mg

Zesty Turkey Loaf

2 pounds ground uncooked turkey
3 slices rye or whole-wheat bread, torn up
2 egg whites
1 onion, finely diced
2 teaspoons prepared white horseradish
1 teaspoon dry mustard
½ cup unsalted tomato sauce

Combine ground turkey with torn bits of bread. Add egg whites, onion, horseradish, and mustard. Add tomato sauce. Mix well, breaking down the bread bits as you go. Place in a 9 × 5–inch nonstick loaf pan. Bake in a 375° F oven for 1¼ hours.

SERVES: 8
CALORIES PER SERVING: 181

NUTRITION PER SERVING

Carbohydrate: .... 6 g	Cholesterol: .... 58 mg	Potassium: .... 432 mg
Protein: .... 30 g	Fiber: .... .3 g	Calcium: .... 14 mg
Total Fat: .... 3.4 g	Sodium: .... 132 mg	Iron: .... 1.4 mg

Turkey Banana Loaf

1 pound ground turkey
1 ripe banana, mashed
1/2 cup uncooked oatmeal
1 egg white
1 tablespoon chopped parsley
1/4 teaspoon pepper
1/4 teaspoon dried thyme

Combine turkey, banana, oatmeal, and egg white until well blended. Add parsley, pepper, and thyme. Pack into a 8 × 4–inch loaf pan. Bake in a 350° F oven for 1 hour.

SERVES: 6

CALORIES PER SERVING: 163

NUTRITION PER SERVING

Carbohydrate: .... 6 g	Cholesterol: .... 21 mg	Potassium: .... 408 mg
Protein: .... 26 g	Fiber: .... .2 g	Calcium: .... 5 mg
Total Fat: .... 3 g	Sodium: .... 114 mg	Iron: .... 1.2 mg

Oatmeal Turkey Loaf

1 pound ground turkey
1/2 cup uncooked oatmeal
1 egg white
1 can (8 ounce) tomato sauce
1 small onion, grated
1 tablespoon grated Parmesan cheese
1 tablespoon chopped parsley
1/2 teaspoon garlic powder
1/4 teaspoon pepper

Combine turkey, oatmeal, egg white, 1/4 cup of the tomato sauce, grated onion, cheese, parsley, garlic powder, and pepper. Mix well. Spoon into a loaf pan. Top with remaining tomato sauce. Bake in a 350° F oven for 1 hour.

SERVES: 6

CALORIES PER SERVING: 166

NUTRITION PER SERVING

Carbohydrate: ...... 5.6 g	Cholesterol: .... 22 mg	Potassium: .... 493 mg
Protein: .... 27 g	Fiber: .... .4 g	Calcium: .... 26 mg
Total Fat: .... 3.3 g	Sodium: .... 124 mg	Iron: .... 1.4 mg

Baked Spinach Balls

1½ pounds ground turkey
1 large onion, finely chopped
1 package (10 ounce) frozen chopped spinach, thawed
1 egg white
¼ teaspoon garlic powder
¼ teaspoon pepper
1 can (16 ounce) unsalted tomato sauce
¼ cup dry red wine
1 cup salt-free chicken broth (see p. 185)
1 tablespoon cornstarch

Combine turkey, onion, thawed chopped spinach, egg white, garlic powder, and pepper. Mix well. Form into 1-inch balls. Place in a heavy saucepan. Combine tomato sauce, red wine, and chicken broth; pour over spinach balls. Cover tightly and cook over low heat 45 minutes. Stir cornstarch and a small amount of water together to make a thin, lump-free paste; add several spoons of hot sauce from meatballs, then return all to the pot, stirring constantly. Cook and stir until sauce thickens. Serve over hot cooked rice or noodles, if desired.

SERVES: 4
CALORIES PER SERVING: 252

NUTRITION PER SERVING

Carbohydrate: .... 31 g	Cholesterol: .... 77 mg	Potassium: .... 950 mg
Protein: .... 40 g	Fiber: .... 1 g	Calcium: .... 63 mg
Total Fat: .... 4.5 g	Sodium: .... 133 mg	Iron: .... 3 mg

Turkey Balls Ratatouille

1 pound raw ground turkey
1 small onion, grated
2 tablespoons chopped parsley
2 slices whole-wheat bread
1 can (6 ounce) salt-free tomato paste
½ cup water
1 clove garlic, minced
1 onion, thinly sliced
1 medium eggplant, peeled and diced into 1-inch cubes
2 zucchini, sliced
1 green pepper, seeded and diced
4 tomatoes, chopped
¼ teaspoon dried thyme
¼ teaspoon dried oregano
⅛ teaspoon pepper

Combine ground turkey, onion, and parsley. Soak bread in water and shred over mixture. Mix well. Form into 1-inch balls. Place in a large skillet. Combine contents of can of tomato paste with water; pour over turkey balls. Add garlic, onion, eggplant, zucchini, green pepper, tomatoes, thyme, oregano, and pepper. Cover and cook over low heat for 30 minutes.

SERVES: 4
CALORIES PER SERVING: 325

NUTRITION PER SERVING

Carbohydrate: ....27 g	Cholesterol: .... 31 mg	Potassium: ..... 1,296 mg
Protein:.............42 g	Fiber: ....3 g	Calcium:.......... 76 mg
Total Fat: ....5 g	Sodium: ....207 mg	Iron: .... 3.8 mg

——6——

Pasta Entrées

Pasta with Shrimp Yogurt Sauce

8 ounces pasta twists
3 quarts boiling water
1 cup plain lowfat yogurt
16 large cooked peeled shrimp
1 tablespoon sliced scallions
2 tablespoons chopped fresh parsley
¼ teaspoon Worcestershire sauce

Cook pasta in boiling water 9–12 minutes until tender; drain. Combine yogurt, 4 shrimp, scallions, parsley, and Worcestershire sauce in a blender. Cover and blend until almost smooth. Serve over hot pasta. Add remaining whole-cooked shrimp and toss.

SERVES: 4

CALORIES PER SERVING: 244

NUTRITION PER SERVING

Carbohydrate: ....37 g	Cholesterol: .... 89 mg	Potassium: ....384 mg
Protein:.............19 g	Fiber: ....1 g	Calcium:.........168 mg
Total Fat: .... 1.7 g	Sodium: .... 90 mg	Iron: .... 2.5 mg

Linguini with Vegetable Garlic Sauce

4 ounces linguini
1½ quarts boiling water
1 tablespoon olive oil
1 clove garlic, minced
1 cup zucchini, sliced thin
1 cup diagonally sliced celery
1 green pepper, cut in strips
¼ teaspoon dried basil
⅛ teaspoon pepper
½ cup cherry tomatoes

Cook linguini in boiling water 9–12 minutes, until tender; drain. Meanwhile, heat olive oil in a wok or nonstick skillet. Add garlic, zucchini, celery, green pepper, basil, and pepper; stir-fry about 5 minutes, until vegetables are tender but still crisp. Add tomatoes and cook for several minutes more. Serve over cooked linguini.

SERVES: 2

CALORIES PER SERVING: 267

NUTRITION PER SERVING

Carbohydrate: .... 46 g	Cholesterol: .... none	Potassium: .... 755 mg
Protein: .... 7 g	Fiber: .... 2.1 g	Calcium: .... 73 mg
Total Fat: .... 7 g	Sodium: .... 61 mg	Iron: .... 2.6 mg

Baked Macaroni and Spinach

8 ounces macaroni
3 quarts boiling water
2 cups unsalted tomato sauce
1 package (10 ounce) frozen chopped spinach, thawed
1 tablespoon grated onion
1 cup skim milk ricotta cheese
¼ teaspoon nutmeg
⅛ teaspoon pepper

Cook macaroni in boiling water 9–12 minutes until tender; drain. Spoon a layer of tomato sauce into a small nonstick baking dish. Then spoon half the macaroni over the bottom of the baking dish. Top with a mixture of spinach, onion, ricotta cheese, nutmeg, and pepper. Spoon remaining macaroni over top. Pour remaining sauce over all. Bake in a 350° F oven 20 minutes, or until heated through.

SERVES: 4

CALORIES PER SERVING: 276

NUTRITION PER SERVING

Carbohydrate: .... 43 g	Cholesterol: .... 19 mg	Potassium: .... 612 mg
Protein:............ 14 g	Fiber: .... 1.1 g	Calcium:......... 236 mg
Total Fat: .... 6 g	Sodium: .... 28 mg	Iron: .... 3.2 mg

Baked Macaroni and Cottage Cheese

4 ounces elbow macaroni
1½ quarts boiling water
1 egg white
½ cup skim milk
¾ cup 1% lowfat cottage cheese
½ teaspoon Worcestershire sauce
⅓ cup chopped onion
⅓ chopped celery
1 tablespoon chopped fresh parsley

Cook macaroni in boiling water for 8 minutes, or until just tender. Beat egg white, add milk, and stir mixture into cottage cheese. Add Worcestershire sauce, onion, celery, and parsley. Stir mixture through cooked macaroni. Pour into a greased casserole and bake in a 350° F oven for 35 minutes, or until lightly browned.

SERVES: 2

CALORIES PER SERVING: 260

NUTRITION PER SERVING

Carbohydrate: .... 41 g	Cholesterol: .... 5 mg	Potassium: .... 406 mg
Protein:............ 10 g	Fiber: .... .4 g	Calcium:......... 159 mg
Total Fat: .... 2 g	Sodium: .... 86 mg	Iron: .... 1.7 mg

Macaroni Stuffed Eggplant

1 medium eggplant
1 small onion, diced
2 stalks celery, sliced
½ cup unsalted tomato juice
¼ teaspoon oregano
1 cup cooked macaroni
1 tablespoon grated Parmesan cheese

Cut eggplant in half and scoop out flesh carefully, leaving the shells unbroken. Dice scooped out eggplant; place in a saucepan with onion, celery, tomato juice, and oregano; simmer until tender. Remove from heat; add cooked macaroni, and spoon mixture into eggplant shells. Top with a sprinkling of grated cheese. Bake 20 minutes in a 350° F oven.

SERVES: 2

CALORIES PER SERVING: 134

NUTRITION PER SERVING

Carbohydrate: ....25 g	Cholesterol: .... 2 mg	Potassium: ....494 mg
Protein:..............6 g	Fiber: .... 1.5 g	Calcium:.......... 84 mg
Total Fat: .... 1.5 g	Sodium: .... 152 mg	Iron: .... 2 mg

Eggplant Lasagna

1 medium eggplant, peeled and diced
4 fresh tomatoes, diced
2 stalks celery, sliced
1 small onion, diced
1 clove garlic, diced
1 tablespoon chopped parsley
½ teaspoon dried basil
9 lasagna noodles
1 quart boiling water
½ cup unsalted tomato juice
¼ cup finely diced skim-milk mozzarella cheese

Cook eggplant, tomatoes, celery, onion, garlic, parsley, and basil in a nonstick skillet, stirring frequently, about 10 minutes. Meanwhile, cook lasagna noodles in boiling water until almost tender; drain and rinse to keep noodles separate. Place 3 noodles side by side in a greased 9 × 13–inch baking dish. Top with a layer of half the eggplant mixture, then another layer of 3 noodles, then another layer of the remaining eggplant mixture, and finally the last 3 noodles. Pour tomato juice over all. Sprinkle with diced mozzarella cheese. Bake in a 350° F oven for 25 minutes.

SERVES: 4
CALORIES PER SERVING: 225

NUTRITION PER SERVING

Carbohydrate: .... 43 g	Cholesterol: .... 3 mg	Potassium: .... 623 mg
Protein: .... 8 g	Fiber: .... 1.5 g	Calcium: .... 130 mg
Total Fat: .... 2 g	Sodium: .... 32 mg	Iron: .... 2.6 mg

Apple Raisin Noodle Pudding

8 ounces wide noodles, cooked and drained
2 apples, peeled, cored, thinly sliced
2 tablespoons lemon juice
¹/₂ teaspoon ground cinnamon
1 cup 1% lowfat cottage cheese
2 tablespoons frozen apple-juice concentrate
¹/₄ cup seedless white raisins
1 egg white

Combine cooked noodles with sliced apples, lemon juice, and cinnamon. Separately, combine cottage cheese, apple-juice concentrate, and raisins. Beat egg white until soft peaks form; fold through cottage cheese mixture. Fold cheese through noodle mixture. Spoon into a 8 × 12–inch nonstick baking pan. Bake in a 350° F oven for 35 minutes, or until top is lightly browned.

SERVES: 6

CALORIES PER SERVING: 216

NUTRITION PER SERVING

Carbohydrate: .... 39 g	Cholesterol: ...... 1.7 mg	Potassium: .... 205 mg
Protein: .... 10 g	Fiber: .... .7 g	Calcium: .... 43 mg
Total Fat: .... 2 g	Sodium: .... 12 mg	Iron: .... 1.4 mg

Baked Noodles and Broccoli

1 package (8 ounce) wide noodles, cooked, drained
1 pound fresh broccoli, cooked, chopped
1 cup skim ricotta cheese
3 scallions, including tops, thinly sliced
1 egg white, beaten
¼ cup whole-wheat bread crumbs
2 tablespoons grated Parmesan cheese

Combine cooked noodles and broccoli. Separately, combine ricotta cheese, scallions, and egg white; add the noodle-broccoli mixture and toss lightly to mix through. Spoon into a nonstick baking dish. Top with bread crumbs and sprinkle with grated cheese. Bake in a 350° F oven for 30 minutes.

SERVES: 4

CALORIES PER SERVING: 304

NUTRITION PER SERVING

Carbohydrate: .... 44 g	Cholesterol: .... 21 mg	Potassium: .... 426 mg
Protein: .... 18 g	Fiber: .... 1.5 g	Calcium: .... 308 mg
Total Fat: .... 7 g	Sodium: .... 90 mg	Iron: .... 2.5 mg

Lasagna Florentine

9 lasagna noodles
1 quart boiling water
1 tablespoon vegetable oil
½ pound fresh mushrooms, sliced
2 medium onions, finely diced
2 cloves garlic, finely minced
1 pound fresh spinach, washed and trimmed
2 cups coarsely chopped fresh carrots
1 cup skim-milk ricotta cheese
1 egg white
1 can (8 ounce) unsalted tomato sauce
3 tablespoons grated Parmesan cheese

Cook noodles in boiling water until almost tender. Drain and rinse to keep separate. Heat oil in a large saucepan; sauté mushrooms, onions, and garlic, stirring to keep them from sticking. Add spinach, torn into small bits, and chopped carrots. Cook until spinach is tender, 2–3 minutes, stirring constantly. Combine ricotta cheese and egg white, beating well; add to spinach mixture. Pour a thin layer of tomato sauce over the bottom of a 13 × 9–inch baking dish. Arrange 3 lasagna noodles in dish over sauce. Spread half the spinach mixture in a thin layer over noodles. Sprinkle with 1 tablespoon Parmesan cheese. Top with 3 more lasagna noodles, spread remaining spinach mixture, and sprinkle with 1 tablespoon Parmesan cheese. Arrange final 3 lasagna noodles over top. Pour remaining tomato sauce over all. Sprinkle with remaining tablespoon of Parmesan cheese.. Bake in a 375° F oven 25 minutes. Let stand 10 to 15 minutes before cutting.

SERVES: 6

CALORIES PER SERVING: 220

NUTRITION PER SERVING

Carbohydrate: ....33 g	Cholesterol: .... 15 mg	Potassium: .... 528 mg
Protein:.............12 g	Fiber: ....1 g	Calcium:.........206 mg
Total Fat: .... 4.7 g	Sodium: .... 68 mg	Iron: .... 2.4 mg

Zucchini Lasagna

8 ounces lasagna noodles
¼ cup water
1 onion, chopped fine
1 clove garlic, minced
1 green pepper, chopped fine
3 cups chopped tomatoes
¼ teaspoon pepper
½ teaspoon dried oregano
1 large zucchini, sliced paper-thin lengthwise
2 cups skim-milk ricotta cheese
1 egg white
½ cup shredded sapsago cheese

Cook lasagna noodles until pliable but still firm; rinse under cold water and drain well. Meanwhile, heat water in a large skillet. Add onion, garlic, green pepper, tomatoes, pepper, and oregano. Cover and simmer 10 minutes. Spread a thin layer of this sauce over the bottom of a rectangular baking dish. Top with a layer of zucchini, then a layer of cooked lasagna noodles. Beat ricotta cheese and egg white together; spread half of this mixture over the noodles. Sprinkle with half of the sapsago cheese. Add another layer of noodles over this; top with remaining cheese mixture and then a layer of noodles. Top with a final layer of zucchini. Spread remaining sauce over top. Sprinkle with remaining sapsago cheese. Bake in a 350° F oven for 30 minutes.

SERVES: 6
CALORIES PER SERVING: 142

NUTRITION PER SERVING

Carbohydrate: ..... 20.5 g	Cholesterol: .... 4 mg	Potassium: .... 43 mg
Protein:............14 g	Fiber: .... 1.1 g	Calcium:.......... 57 mg
Total Fat: .... 1.5 g	Sodium: .... 118 mg	Iron: .... 1.4 mg

Stuffed Baked Manicotti

1 pound manicotti pasta tubes
3 quarts boiling water
3 cups skim-milk ricotta cheese
¼ cup sliced scallions, including green tops
1 can (16 ounce) tomatoes
2 tablespoons tomato paste
½ teaspoon oregano
¼ teaspoon basil
¼ teaspoon pepper
½ cup whole-wheat bread crumbs

Cook manicotti in boiling water until pliable, about 7 minutes. Combine ricotta cheese and scallions; stuff manicotti tubes with the mixture and place side by side in a nonstick flat casserole. Blend tomatoes, tomato paste, oregano, basil, and pepper; spoon over stuffed manicotti. Top with bread crumbs. Bake in a 350° F oven for 30 minutes.

SERVES: 6
CALORIES PER SERVING: 240
NUTRITION PER SERVING
Carbohydrate: ....35 g	Cholesterol: .... 5 mg	Potassium: ....396 mg
Protein:.............19 g	Fiber: ....6 g	Calcium:.......... 95 mg
Total Fat: .... 2.1 g	Sodium: .... 167 mg	Iron: .... 1.8 mg

Pasta Bow Ties with Yogurt Mushroom Sauce

¼ pound fresh sliced mushrooms
1 onion, diced
½ cup salt-free chicken broth (see page 185)
¼ cup plain nonfat yogurt
⅛ teaspoon pepper
¼ teaspoon dried dillweed
4 ounces pasta bow ties
1½ quarts boiling water

Cook mushrooms and onion in a nonstick skillet for a few minutes until limp, stirring frequently. Add chicken broth; cook uncovered until liquid reduces by half. Remove from heat; stir in yogurt, pepper, and dillweed. Meanwhile, cook pasta bow ties in boiling water until tender, about 8 minutes; drain. Toss with mushroom sauce and serve.

SERVES: 2
CALORIES PER SERVING: 193

NUTRITION PER SERVING

Carbohydrate: .... 38 g	Cholesterol: .... .5 mg	Potassium: .... 355 mg
Protein: .... 8 g	Fiber: .... .5 g	Calcium: .... 55 mg
Total Fat: .... 1 g	Sodium: .... 10 mg	Iron: .... 1.8 mg

Rigatoni with Hot Chili Sauce

1 onion, diced
½ teaspoon dried chili peppers
1 clove garlic, finely minced
½ teaspoon chili powder
1 can (8 ounce) tomato sauce
4 ounces rigatoni
1½ quarts boiling water
2 tablespoons grated Romano cheese
dash of pepper

Sauté onion, chili peppers, and garlic in a nonstick skillet, stirring frequently, until onion is limp. Add chili powder and tomato sauce. Cover and simmer for 10 minutes. Meanwhile, cook rigatoni in boiling water for 9–12 minutes, or until tender; drain. Toss rigatoni with sauce. Serve with grated cheese and a dash of pepper.

SERVES: 2

CALORIES PER SERVING: 220

NUTRITION PER SERVING

Carbohydrate: ....41 g	Cholesterol: .... 5 mg	Potassium: ....444 mg
Protein:..............9 g	Fiber: ....9 g	Calcium:.........119 mg
Total Fat: ....3 g	Sodium: ....53 mg	Iron: .... 2.1 mg

Spaghetti with Tomato Cucumber Sauce

4 ounces spaghetti
1½ quarts boiling water
1½ cups coarsely chopped fresh tomatoes
¾ cup coarsely chopped, seeded, pared cucumber
1 small clove garlic
¼ teaspoon dried oregano
⅛ teaspoon pepper

Cook spaghetti in boiling water 9–12 minutes until tender; drain. Meanwhile, place half of the tomatoes and cucumber, garlic, oregano, and pepper in a blender; process until smooth. Add rest of tomatoes and cucumber to the puree and pour over cooked spaghetti.

SERVES: 2

CALORIES PER SERVING: 277

NUTRITION PER SERVING

Carbohydrate: . . . . 45 g	Cholesterol: . . . . none	Potassium: . . . . 738 mg
Protein: . . . . 7 g	Fiber: . . . . 1.7 g	Calcium: . . . . 50 mg
Total Fat: . . . . 1 g	Sodium: . . . . 11 mg	Iron: . . . . 2.8 mg

Vegetable Pasta Casserole

4 ounces spaghetti
1½ quarts boiling water
½ cup 1% lowfat cottage cheese
½ cup plain nonfat yogurt
1 cup cooked cut green beans
1 cup cooked sliced carrots
¼ teaspoon dried dillweed
⅛ teaspoon pepper

Cook spaghetti in boiling water for 9 minutes; drain. Combine cottage cheese and yogurt. Place half the spaghetti in a nonstick flat baking dish, top with half the cheese mixture, then with a layer of beans topped with carrots. Sprinkle with dillweed and pepper. Spread with remaining cheese mixture and top with second half of spaghetti. Bake in a 350° F oven for 30 minutes.

SERVES: 2

CALORIES PER SERVING: 268

NUTRITION PER SERVING

Carbohydrate: . . . . 47 g	Cholesterol: . . . . 3 mg	Potassium: . . . . 545 mg
Protein: . . . . 17 g	Fiber: . . . . 1.5 g	Calcium: . . . . 215 mg
Total Fat: . . . . 1.5 g	Sodium: . . . . 29 mg	Iron: . . . . 2.3 mg

Meatless Spaghetti Sauce

1 can (35 ounce) unsalted Italian tomatoes in sauce
1 can (6 ounce) unsalted tomato paste
1 onion, finely diced
½ teaspoon dried basil
½ teaspoon dried oregano

Empty tomatoes and tomato paste into a large saucepan. Add onion, basil, and oregano. Cover and simmer over low heat for 30 minutes. Mash tomatoes into a puree, using a slotted spoon or potato masher. Use as a sauce for pasta. Makes 5 cups of sauce.

SERVES: 10 (½-Cup Servings)
CALORIES PER SERVING: 28

NUTRITION PER SERVING

Carbohydrate: .... 7 g	Cholesterol: .... none	Potassium: .... 313 mg
Protein: .... 1 g	Fiber: .... .7 g	Calcium: .... 18 mg
Total Fat: .... trace	Sodium: .... 5 mg	Iron: .... .6 mg

7

Rice and Other Grains

Brown Rice Español

1 cup short-grain brown rice
2½ cups water
1 cup chopped tomatoes
1 green pepper, finely diced
1 onion, finely diced
2 tablespoons chopped fresh parsley
⅛ teaspoon pepper

Place rice and water in a saucepan; bring to a boil. Stir. Cover and cook for 40 minutes, fluffing once with a fork. Rice should be tender and water evaporated when done. Meanwhile, cook tomatoes, green pepper, onion, parsley, and pepper together in a saucepan. Toss tomato mixture through cooked rice and serve.

SERVES: 6
CALORIES PER SERVING: 125

NUTRITION PER SERVING

Carbohydrate: .... 28 g	Cholesterol: .... none	Potassium: .... 135 mg
Protein: .... 2.6 g	Fiber: .... .75 g	Calcium: .... 20 mg
Total Fat: .... trace	Sodium: .... 388 mg	Iron: .... 1.2 mg

Baked Rice and Peas Amandine

1 cup chopped onions
1 cup chopped celery
½ cup sliced mushrooms
2½ cups salt-free chicken broth (see page 185)
1 cup brown rice
¾ teaspoon poultry seasoning
1 cup green peas, fresh or frozen
2 tablespoons slivered almonds

Simmer onions, celery, and mushrooms in ½ cup of the chicken broth in a nonstick skillet, until vegetables are tender. Pour into a 2-quart nonstick baking dish. Add rice, remaining broth, poultry seasoning, and peas. Cover and bake in a 350° F oven for 40 minutes, or until rice is tender and liquid is absorbed. Fluff with a fork. Spoon into a serving dish and sprinkle with almonds.

SERVES: 8
CALORIES PER SERVING: 121

NUTRITION PER SERVING

Carbohydrate: .... 23 g	Cholesterol: .... none	Potassium: .... 194 mg
Protein: .... 4 g	Fiber: .... 1.2 g	Calcium: .... 28 mg
Total Fat: .... 1.5 g	Sodium: .... 47 mg	Iron: .... 1 mg

Orange Rice

1 cup brown rice
1 cup orange juice
1½ cups water
½ teaspoon dried dillweed
¼ cup sliced scallions

Combine rice, orange juice, water, and dillweed in a large saucepan. Add scallions. Bring to a boil, then turn the heat low and cover tightly. Simmer over low heat for 40 minutes, stirring once during the cooking time. Add additional water if needed.

SERVES: 6
CALORIES PER SERVING: 132

NUTRITION PER SERVING

Carbohydrate: ....29 g	Cholesterol: .... none	Potassium: ....160 mg
Protein:..............4 g	Fiber: ....8 g	Calcium:..........16 mg
Total Fat: ....5 g	Sodium: ....3 mg	Iron: ....6 mg

Brown Rice Cucumber Salad

3 cups cold cooked brown rice
¼ pound sliced fresh mushrooms
¼ cup sliced green onions, including tops
1 large cucumber, peeled, seeded and diced
½ cup sliced celery
1 tomato coarsely chopped
1 cup cold cooked peas
¼ cup chopped fresh parsley
2 tablespoons olive oil
2 tablespoons red wine vinegar
¼ teaspoon dry mustard

Combine rice, mushrooms, onions, cucumber, celery, tomato, peas, and parsley in a large bowl. Mix well. Separately, stir together oil, vinegar, and mustard; pour over salad and toss well. Chill at least 2 hours before serving.

SERVES: 6
CALORIES PER SERVING: 184

NUTRITION PER SERVING

Carbohydrate: ....30 g	Cholesterol: .... none	Potassium: ....250 mg
Protein:..............6 g	Fiber: ....1.6 g	Calcium:..........33 mg
Total Fat: ....4.8 g	Sodium: ....322 mg	Iron: ....1.4 mg

Kasha Tabbouleh

1 cup cooked kasha (whole, coarse, or medium)
⅓ cup chopped scallions
¼ cup chopped fresh parsley
1 teaspoon dried mint leaves
1 large tomato, seeded and chopped
1 tablespoon lemon juice
1 tablespoon olive oil
2 teaspoons red wine vinegar
⅛ teaspoon pepper
8 romaine lettuce leaves

Combine all ingredients except the lettuce leaves. Chill for at least 2 hours before serving. Place tabbouleh in a mound in the center of the plate and surround it with romaine lettuce leaves. Serve as an appetizer or salad course.

SERVES: 4
CALORIES PER SERVING: 102

NUTRITION PER SERVING

Carbohydrate: .... 16 g	Cholesterol: .... none	Potassium: .... 233 mg
Protein: .... 2 g	Fiber: .... .9 g	Calcium: .... 38 mg
Total Fat: .... 3.5 g	Sodium: .... 8 mg	Iron: .... 1.1 mg

Baked Kasha and Zucchini

1½ cups kasha (buckwheat groats)
2 medium zucchini, coarsely grated
1 onion, finely diced
¼ teaspoon pepper
¼ teaspoon dried thyme
¼ cup grated sapsago cheese

Cook kasha according to package directions. Meanwhile, place grated zucchini, onion, pepper, and thyme in a nonstick skillet. Add ¼ cup water. Cover and cook over low heat 4 minutes. Combine with cooked kasha. Spoon into a nonstick baking dish. Top with grated sapsago cheese. Bake 15 minutes in a preheated 350° F oven.

SERVES: 6
CALORIES PER SERVING: 113

NUTRITION PER SERVING

Carbohydrate: 23 g	Cholesterol: 3 mg	Potassium: 205 mg
Protein: 3.5 g	Fiber: .6 g	Calcium: 51 mg
Total Fat: 1 g	Sodium: 2 mg	Iron: .6 mg

──8──
Vegetables

Creole Green Beans

1 pound green beans, trimmed
2 tomatoes, chopped
½ green pepper, finely diced
½ small onion, finely diced
1 okra pod, thinly sliced (optional)
¼ cup water
⅛ teaspoon thyme
⅛ teaspoon pepper

Wash green beans and place wet in a medium saucepan. Add remaining ingredients. Cover and cook over low heat until beans are tender, about 10 to 15 minutes.

SERVES: 6
CALORIES PER SERVING: 23

NUTRITION PER SERVING

Carbohydrate: .... 5 g	Cholesterol: .... none	Potassium: .... 190 mg
Protein: .... 1 g	Fiber: .... .8 g	Calcium: 31mg
Total Fat: .... trace	Sodium: .... 4 mg	Iron: .... .6 mg

Creole Lentils

½ cup dried lentils
1 tablespoon olive oil
1 green pepper, seeded, finely chopped
1 onion, finely chopped
2 tomatoes, finely chopped
⅛ teaspoon pepper
⅛ teaspoon thyme
⅛ teaspoon filé powder (optional)
2 cups cooked brown rice

Cover lentils with water and soak overnight. Drain, cover with fresh water, and cook over low heat, covered, until lentils are tender, about 1 hour. Heat olive oil in a nonstick skillet; sauté green pepper and onion until limp. Add tomatoes, pepper, thyme, and filé powder. Cook 5 minutes. Drain lentils and add to tomatoes; simmer, covered, 5 minutes more. Serve over cooked brown rice.

SERVES: 4
CALORIES PER SERVING: 222

NUTRITION PER SERVING

Carbohydrate: . . . . 40 g	Cholesterol: . . . . none	Potassium: . . . . 416 mg
Protein: . . . . 78 g	Fiber: . . . . 2 g	Calcium: . . . . 39 mg
Total Fat: . . . . 3.7 g	Sodium: . . . . 282 mg	Iron: . . . . 2.1 mg

Broccoli Polonaise

1 pound fresh broccoli
½ cup chopped fresh mushrooms
¼ cup salt-free tomato juice
1 tablespoon fresh lemon juice
½ cup grated carrots
¼ cup bread crumbs
1 tablespoon grated lemon rind

Trim broccoli and wash well. Drain. Cut in half or in quarters the long way, depending on thickness of stems. Cook in a small amount of water, or steam, until tender. Drain. Meanwhile, in a small skillet, cook mushrooms in tomato juice until limp. Add lemon juice, carrots, bread crumbs, and lemon rind. Stir and heat through. Spoon over cooked broccoli and serve.

SERVES: 4

CALORIES PER SERVING: 64

NUTRITION PER SERVING

Carbohydrate: ....12 g	Cholesterol: .... none	Potassium: ....444 mg
Protein:..............5 g	Fiber: ....2 g	Calcium:..........97 mg
Total Fat: ....7 g	Sodium: ....65 mg	Iron: .... 1.3 mg

Baked Stuffed Butternut Squash

2 small butternut squash
¹/₂ cup grated carrots
¹/₄ cup white seedless raisins
¹/₄ cup frozen apple-juice concentrate
¹/₈ teaspoon ginger
¹/₈ teaspoon nutmeg

Cut butternut squash in halves the long way. Scoop out seeds and discard. Combine carrots, raisins, apple-juice concentrate, ginger, and nutmeg. Stuff squash cavities with this mixture. Place squash halves in a baking pan. Bake uncovered, in a 350° F oven for 40 minutes, or until fork-tender.

SERVES: 4

CALORIES PER SERVING: 119

NUTRITION PER SERVING

Carbohydrate: ....30 g	Cholesterol: .... none	Potassium: ....636 mg
Protein:............ 2.5 g	Fiber: ....2 g	Calcium:..........42 mg
Total Fat: ....5 g	Sodium: ....10 mg	Iron: .... 1.5 mg

Wheat-Germ Slaw

1 small head cabbage, shredded
1 large carrot, grated
½ cup wheat germ
¼ cup sliced green onion, including tops
¼ cup chopped fresh parsley
1 cup plain nonfat yogurt
¼ teaspoon dry mustard
½ teaspoon dried dillweed
¼ teaspoon celery seed

Combine cabbage, carrot, wheat germ, green onion, and parsley. Separately, mix yogurt, mustard, dillweed, and celery seed together; pour over cabbage mixture. Toss well. Refrigerate until ready to serve.

SERVES: 8
CALORIES PER SERVING: 53

NUTRITION PER SERVING

Carbohydrate: .... 8 g	Cholesterol: .... .5 mg	Potassium: .... 260 mg
Protein: .... 4 g	Fiber: .... .6 g	Calcium: .... 84 mg
Total Fat: .... 1 g	Sodium: .... 12 mg	Iron: .... .9 mg

Cole Slaw with Roquefort Dressing

6 cups shredded cabbage
½ cup grated carrot
2 tablespoons grated onion
1 cup plain nonfat yogurt
2 tablespoons wine vinegar
2 tablespoons Roquefort cheese, crumbled
1 tablespoon sugar
¼ teaspoon pepper
½ teaspoon celery seed

In a large bowl, combine cabbage, carrot, and onion. Separately, combine yogurt, vinegar, cheese, sugar, pepper, and celery seed; pour over cabbage and toss well. Refrigerate for several hours until ready to serve.

SERVES: 10

CALORIES PER SERVING: 39

NUTRITION PER SERVING

Carbohydrate: .... 6 g	Cholesterol: ...... 2.5 mg	Potassium: .... 185 mg
Protein: .... 2.6 g	Fiber: .... .4 g	Calcium: .... 83 mg
Total Fat: .... .8 g	Sodium: .... 11 mg	Iron: .... .3 mg

Carrot Slaw

1 small cabbage, sliced thin
2 cups thinly sliced celery
1 cup coarsely shredded carrots
1 green pepper, seeded, thinly sliced
2 tablespoons cider vinegar
½ teaspoon white pepper
1 teaspoon honey
½ teaspoon celery seed
1 cup plain nonfat yogurt

In a large bowl, combine cabbage, celery, carrots, and slices of pepper. Stir vinegar, white pepper, honey, and celery seed into yogurt; pour over vegetables and mix well. Chill.

SERVES: 8

CALORIES PER SERVING: 38

NUTRITION PER SERVING

Carbohydrate: .... 8 g	Cholesterol: .... .5 mg	Potassium: .... 327 mg
Protein: .... 3 g	Fiber: .... .7 g	Calcium: .... 91 mg
Total Fat: .... trace	Sodium: .... 52 mg	Iron: .... .5 mg

Carrot Stuffed Baked Potato

2 baking potatoes
½ cup skim milk
2 soft-cooked carrots
¼ teaspoon dillweed
2 tablespoons grated sapsago cheese

Scrub potatoes and bake 1 hour in a 350° F oven. Remove from oven. Cut potatoes in half the long way. Scoop out cooked potato, reserving skin shells. Mash with milk, carrots, and dillweed. Spoon mixture back into reserved potato shells. Top with grated cheese. Return to oven to melt cheese and heat through.

SERVES: 4
CALORIES PER SERVING: 103

NUTRITION PER SERVING

Carbohydrate: .... 22 g	Cholesterol: .... .7 mg	Potassium: .... 571 mg
Protein: .... 4 g	Fiber: .... .4 g	Calcium: .... 62 mg
Total Fat: .... trace	Sodium: .... 36 mg	Iron: .... .8 mg

Collards Parmesan

2 pounds fresh collard greens
1 clove garlic, crushed
1 tablespoon olive oil
⅛ teaspoon pepper
⅛ teaspoon nutmeg
2 tablespoons grated Parmesan cheese
6 thinly sliced raw red onion rings

Wash and trim collard greens. Mix garlic, oil, pepper, and nutmeg in a large nonstick skillet. Add washed and trimmed collard greens. Cover and cook over low heat until tender, adding a little more water if the water clinging to the washed greens has completely evaporated. Mix lightly with a fork. Turn onto a serving platter and sprinkle with Parmesan cheese. Top with raw red onion rings.

SERVES: 6
CALORIES PER SERVING: 98

NUTRITION PER SERVING

Carbohydrate: .... 11 g	Cholesterol: ...... 1.6 mg	Potassium: .... 518 mg
Protein: .... 8 g	Fiber: .... 2 g	Calcium: .... 388 mg
Total fat: .... 3.8 g	Sodium: .... 16 mg	Iron: .... 1.6 mg

Cranberry Vegetable Mold

2 envelopes (2 tablespoons) unflavored gelatin
2 cups cranberry juice
2 cups apple juice
2 tablespoons lemon juice
1 small onion, grated
1 cup ground fresh cranberries
1 cup grated carrots
1 cup thinly sliced celery

Sprinkle gelatin over ½ cup cranberry juice. Let stand 5 minutes to soften. Stir over low heat until gelatin is dissolved. Add remaining cranberry juice, apple juice, and lemon juice. Blend well. Chill until thickened to the consistency of egg white. Fold in onion, cranberries, carrots, and celery. Pour mixture into a 2-quart mold. Chill until firm. Unmold on crisp salad greens.

SERVES: 10
CALORIES PER SERVING: 70

NUTRITION PER SERVING

Carbohydrate: .... 17 g	Cholesterol: .... none	Potassium: .... 140 mg
Protein: .... 1 g	Fiber: .... .2 g	Calcium: .... 15 mg
Total Fat: .... trace	Sodium: .... 17 mg	Iron: .... .6 mg

Pickled Cucumbers

2 cucumbers, peeled, thinly sliced
1 onion, thinly sliced
1 cup water
¼ cup white vinegar
1 tablespoon frozen apple-juice concentrate
¼ teaspoon white pepper
¼ teaspoon dried dillweed

Place sliced cucumbers and onion in a small deep bowl. Combine water, vinegar, apple-juice concentrate, pepper, and dillweed; pour over cucumbers. Cover tightly and refrigerate for several hours or overnight. Stir occasionally.

SERVES: 6
CALORIES PER SERVING: 11

NUTRITION PER SERVING

Carbohydrate: .... 3 g	Cholesterol: .... none	Potassium: .... 63 mg
Protein:............ .16 g	Fiber: .... .2 g	Calcium:........... 8 mg
Total Fat: .... trace	Sodium: .... 2 mg	Iron: .... .36 mg

Baked Eggplant and Tomatoes

1 eggplant, about 2 pounds
1/2 lemon
1/2 teaspoon oregano
1/8 teaspoon pepper
4 medium tomatoes, chopped
2 ounces skim-milk mozarella cheese

Peel and cut the eggplant in half lengthwise, then slice into 1/4-inch slices. Sauté without fat in a nonstick skillet until browned on each side. Place eggplant in a nonstick baking dish, seasoning with squirts of lemon juice, oregano, and pepper as you layer the slices. Place chopped tomatoes on top, then cover with diced cheese. Bake in a 375° F oven for 20 minutes, or until eggplant is tender.

SERVES: 8

CALORIES PER SERVING: 36

NUTRITION PER SERVING

Carbohydrate: ....5 g	Cholesterol: ...... 3.6 mg	Potassium: ....239 mg
Protein:.............2 g	Fiber: ....9 g	Calcium:..........29 mg
Total Fat: ....9 g	Sodium: ....3 mg	Iron: ....6 mg

Stuffed Eggplant

2 medium eggplants
1 onion, diced
4 stalks celery, diced
1 cup salt-free tomato juice
½ teaspoon oregano
1 egg white
1 cup raisin bran cereal
2 tablespoons grated Parmesan cheese

Cut eggplants in half lengthwise. Scoop out flesh, leaving unbroken shells. Dice scooped out eggplant flesh; place in a saucepan with onion, celery, tomato juice, and oregano. Simmer until vegetables are tender. Remove from heat. Add egg white and raisin bran to mixture in saucepan. Fill eggplant shells with this mixture. Sprinkle with grated Parmesan cheese. Bake in a 350° F oven for 20 minutes.

SERVES: 4

CALORIES PER SERVING: 87

NUTRITION PER SERVING

Carbohydrate: .... 17 g	Cholesterol: ...... 2.5 mg	Potassium: .... 427 mg
Protein: .... 4 g	Fiber: .... 1.5 g	Calcium: .... 81 mg
Total Fat: .... 1.2 g	Sodium: .... 187 mg	Iron: .... 3 mg

Eggplant Parmesan

1 can (16 ounce) salt-free tomatoes
2 tablespoons salt-free tomato paste
1 teaspoon dried oregano
1 eggplant, peeled and sliced thin
1 pound sliced skim-milk mozzarella cheese
¼ cup grated Parmesan cheese

Combine tomatoes, tomato paste, and oregano in an electric blender or food processor. Spoon some of the tomato mixture into a thin layer in a large flat baking dish. Cover with slices of eggplant laid side by side. Top with a layer of sliced mozzarella cheese. Sprinkle 1 tablespoon of Parmesan cheese over all. Repeat a layer of sauce, eggplant, and cheese. Finish with a layer of eggplant, sauce, and remaining Parmesan cheese. Bake in a 350° F oven for 35 minutes, or until eggplant is fork-tender.

SERVES: 8
CALORIES PER SERVING: 79

NUTRITION PER SERVING

Carbohydrate: .... 7 g	Cholesterol: .... 5 mg	Potassium: .... 314 mg
Protein: .... 9 g	Fiber: .... .8 g	Calcium: .... 92 mg
Total Fat: .... 1.5 g	Sodium: .... 26 mg	Iron: .... .7 mg

Endive and Chick Pea Yogurt Salad

½ cup plain nonfat yogurt
½ teaspoon dried dillweed
⅛ teaspoon pepper
2 heads of Belgian endive
1 cup cooked chick peas, may be canned
1 tablespoon chopped pimientos

Combine yogurt, dillweed, and pepper in a small bowl. Run cold water over the endive heads and pat dry with a paper towel. Cut the endives into 4 lengthwise sections each. Place them in a salad bowl. Add chick peas to the center of the bowl. Pour dressing over all. Sprinkle pimientos over the dressing.

SERVES: 4
CALORIES PER SERVING: 74

NUTRITION PER SERVING

Carbohydrate: ....13 g	Cholesterol: .... .5 mg	Potassium: ....307 mg
Protein:..............6 g	Fiber: ....8 g	Calcium:..........90 mg
Total Fat: ....2 g	Sodium: ....5 mg	Iron: ....1.5 mg

Alfalfa Sprout Salad

2 cups torn romaine lettuce leaves
1 cup alfalfa sprouts
2 tomatoes, diced
1 green pepper, seeded, diced
¼ cup diced red onion
¼ cup olive oil
2 tablespoons tarragon vinegar
¼ teaspoon dry mustard
⅛ teaspoon dried oregano

Combine lettuce, alfalfa sprouts, tomatoes, green pepper, and onion in a salad bowl. Beat together oil, vinegar, mustard, and oregano; pour over salad and toss lightly.

SERVES: 6

CALORIES PER SERVING: 102

NUTRITION PER SERVING

Carbohydrate: .... 5 g	Cholesterol: .... none	Potassium: .... 223 mg
Protein: .... 1.6 g	Fiber: .... .7 g	Calcium: .... 25 mg
Total Fat: .... 9 g	Sodium: .... 6 mg	Iron: .... .8 mg

Waldorf Banana Sprout Salad

2 red apples, diced
2 stalks celery, diced
1/4 cup seedless raisins
1/2 cup broken walnut pieces
1 banana, sliced
1/2 cup plain nonfat yogurt
6 lettuce cups
1 cup alfalfa sprouts

Combine diced apples, celery, raisins, walnuts, and banana. Add yogurt and mix through. Place 1/6 the mixture in a mound in each lettuce cup. Surround each with a ring of alfalfa sprouts.

SERVES: 6

CALORIES PER SERVING: 144

NUTRITION PER SERVING

Carbohydrate: .... 20 g	Cholesterol: .... .3 mg	Potassium: .... 320 mg
Protein: .... 4 g	Fiber: .... 1 g	Calcium: .... 66 mg
Total Fat: .... 6.8 g	Sodium: .... 4 mg	Iron: .... 1.1 mg

Spinach Sprout Salad

1 pound fresh spinach leaves, trimmed
¼ cup sliced fresh mushrooms
1 red pepper, seeded, sliced
1 cup mung bean sprouts
¼ cup orange juice
2 tablespoons safflower oil
⅛ teaspoon nutmeg
⅛ teaspoon onion powder

Wash spinach leaves and pat dry with paper toweling. Tear larger pieces into bite-size pieces. Add mushrooms, red pepper, and sprouts. Separately, combine orange juice, oil, nutmeg, and onion powder; mix well and pour over salad. Toss lightly and serve.

SERVES: 4
CALORIES PER SERVING: 88

NUTRITION PER SERVING

Carbohydrate: .... 6 g	Cholesterol: .... none	Potassium: .... 266 mg
Protein: .... 2.7 g	Fiber: .... .7 g	Calcium: .... 34 mg
Total Fat: .... 6.7 g	Sodium: .... 24 mg	Iron: .... 1.3 mg

Baked Lima Beans

2 cups dried lima beans
2 onions, thinly sliced
2 carrots, scraped, finely diced
1 cup chopped tomatoes
1 clove garlic, finely minced
1 cup unsalted tomato juice
½ teaspoon Worcestershire sauce
⅛ teaspoon pepper

Soak lima beans for several hours or overnight. Discard soaking water. Place lima beans in a nonstick baking dish. Add onions, carrots, tomatoes, and garlic. Separately, combine tomato juice, Worcestershire sauce, and pepper; pour over bean mixture. Mix well. Cover tightly with a lid or foil. Bake 2 hours in a 350° F oven, or until beans are tender.

SERVES: 6
CALORIES PER SERVING: 209

NUTRITION PER SERVING

Carbohydrate: ....43 g	Cholesterol: .... none	Potassium: ....504 mg
Protein:..............8 g	Fiber: ....15 g	Calcium:..........59 mg
Total Fat: ....8 g	Sodium: ....15 mg	Iron: ....2.6 mg

Lima Corn Casserole

1 cup dried lima beans
2 cups cooked corn kernels
2 onions, thinly sliced
1 can (28 ounce) tomatoes
1/2 teaspoon paprika
1/4 teaspoon dry mustard
1/4 teaspoon dried rosemary
1/4 cup whole-wheat bread crumbs

Soak lima beans overnight in cold water. Cook over low heat 2 hours, or until beans are soft. Combine cooked lima beans with cooked corn in a 2-quart nonstick baking dish. Combine onions, tomatoes, paprika, mustard, and rosemary; spoon over top of beans and corn. Top with bread crumbs. Bake in a 350° F oven for 30 minutes.

SERVES: 6
CALORIES PER SERVING: 160

NUTRITION PER SERVING

Carbohydrate: ....32 g	Cholesterol: .... none	Potassium: ....751 mg
Protein:..............8 g	Fiber: ....2 g	Calcium:..........39 mg
Total Fat: ....6 g	Sodium: ....191 mg	Iron: ....3 mg

Mashed Potato Puff

6 potatoes, peeled and quartered
1 small onion, sliced
½ teaspoon dried dillweed
¼ cup skim milk
2 egg whites
⅛ teaspoon ground white pepper
⅛ teaspoon paprika

Place potatoes, onion, and dillweed in a heavy saucepan. Add an inch of water, cover, and cook until potatoes are tender, about 20 minutes. Drain, reserving liquid. Mash potatoes and onion, adding skim milk to soften mixture. Beat egg whites until stiff peaks form; fold through potato mixture until well blended. Add pepper. Spoon mixture into a nonstick casserole. Swirl top with a fork. Sprinkle with paprika. Bake 20 minutes in a 350° F oven.

SERVES: 6
CALORIES PER SERVING: 102

NUTRITION PER SERVING

Carbohydrate: . . . . 21 g	Cholesterol: . . . . .2 mg	Potassium: . . . . 432 mg
Protein: . . . . 4 g	Fiber: . . . . .8 g	Calcium: . . . . 25 mg
Total Fat: . . . . trace	Sodium: . . . . 25 mg	Iron: . . . . .7 mg

Potato Carrot Pancakes

1 cup shredded, pared raw white potatoes
1 cup shredded raw carrots
1 small onion, finely chopped
½ cup skim milk
½ cup unbleached flour
2 egg whites, slightly beaten
½ teaspoon dried dillweed
¼ teaspoon pepper

Combine shredded potato, carrots, and onion in a bowl. Add milk and flour. Stir in egg whites, dillweed, and pepper. Mix well. If mixture is too thin, add another tablespoon or two of flour. Drop by tablespoonfuls on a nonstick griddle. Brown on one side, turn and brown other side.

SERVES: 6

CALORIES PER SERVING: 88

NUTRITION PER SERVING

Carbohydrate: ....17 g	Cholesterol: .... .3 mg	Potassium: ....239 mg
Protein:.............4 g	Fiber: .... .4 g	Calcium:..........37 mg
Total Fat: ....16 g	Sodium: ....34 mg	Iron: .... .7 mg

High C Salad

>   1 quart fresh torn spinach leaves
>   1 red pepper, seeded, cut into strips
>   2 tomatoes, cut into wedges
>   1 tablespoon safflower oil
>   1/4 cup orange juice
>   2 tablespoons lemon juice
>   1/2 teaspoon garlic powder
>   1/4 teaspoon celery seed
>   1/8 teaspoon white pepper

Combine spinach, red pepper, and tomatoes in a salad bowl. In a jar, combine salad oil, orange and lemon juices, garlic powder, celery seed, and white pepper. Shake well. Pour over salad and toss.

SERVES: 6

CALORIES PER SERVING: 46

NUTRITION PER SERVING

Carbohydrate: ....5 g	Cholesterol: .... none	Potassium: ....326 mg
Protein:.............2 g	Fiber: .... .6 g	Calcium:..........42 mg
Total Fat: ....2 g	Sodium: ....29 mg	Iron: .... 1.4 mg

Creamed Spinach

>   1 pound fresh spinach
>   1 small onion, grated
>   1/4 teaspoon nutmeg
>   1/8 teaspoon pepper
>   1/2 cup plain nonfat yogurt

259

Wash spinach leaves and trim off roots and stems. Place in a skillet with a small amount of water. Add onion, nutmeg, and pepper. Cook, covered, over low heat, until tender, about 5 minutes. Drain well. Toss with yogurt and serve.

SERVES: 4

CALORIES PER SERVING: 35

NUTRITION PER SERVING

Carbohydrate: .... 5 g	Cholesterol: .... .5 mg	Potassium: .... 348 mg
Protein:.............. 4 g	Fiber: .... .4 g	Calcium:......... 110 mg
Total Fat: .... trace	Sodium: .... 40 mg	Iron: .... 1.8 mg

Spinach Cauliflower Salad

1 quart fresh spinach leaves, washed, trimmed
½ small head cauliflower, broken into flowerets
2 cups sliced celery
¼ pound fresh mushrooms, sliced
1 cup halved cherry tomatoes
¼ cup wine vinegar
1 tablespoon lemon juice
¼ cup orange juice
½ teaspoon dried tarragon
⅛ teaspoon pepper

Combine all vegetables in a large salad bowl. Shake vinegar, lemon juice, orange juice, tarragon, and pepper together in a cruet; pour over salad. Toss and serve.

SERVES: 6

CALORIES PER SERVING: 29

NUTRITION PER SERVING

Carbohydrate: .... 6 g	Cholesterol: .... none	Potassium: .... 383 mg
Protein:............ 2.5 g	Fiber: .... .8 g	Calcium:.......... 48 mg
Total Fat: .... trace	Sodium: .... 47 mg	Iron: .... 1.5 mg

Spinach Salad

1 pound fresh spinach, trimmed
1 clove garlic, crushed
2 tablespoons olive oil
¼ teaspoon brown sugar
⅛ teaspoon pepper
2 tablespoons grated Parmesan cheese
¼ cup sliced red onion rings

Wash spinach well, letting some water cling to the leaves at the last rinsing. Combine garlic, oil, sugar, and pepper in a large skillet. Add wet spinach leaves. Cover and bring to a high heat. Reduce heat and simmer until spinach is wilted and just tender, about 4 minutes. Turn onto a serving plate and sprinkle with cheese and red onion rings.

SERVES: 6
CALORIES PER SERVING: 56

NUTRITION PER SERVING

Carbohydrate: . . . . 2 g	Cholesterol: . . . . . . 1.7 mg	Potassium: . . . . 99 mg
Protein: . . . . 1.7 g	Fiber: . . . . .1 g	Calcium: . . . . 47 mg
Total Fat: . . . . 5 g	Sodium: . . . . 29 mg	Iron: . . . . .6 mg

Yolkless Spinach Frittata

½ pound fresh trimmed spinach, or 10 ounces frozen spinach
½ pound fresh mushrooms, sliced
1 small onion, diced fine
1 tablespoon olive oil
4 egg whites
⅛ teaspoon pepper
⅛ teaspoon dried dillweed
2 teaspoons grated Parmesan cheese

Cook spinach in a small amount of water. Drain well. Sauté mushrooms and onion with olive oil in a large nonstick skillet, until limp. Beat egg whites until soft peaks form. Stir in drained spinach, pepper, and dillweed; mix well. Pour mixture over mushrooms and onions in the skillet. Cook over medium heat until mixture is set. Sprinkle with grated Parmesan cheese. Broil until cheese melts and top is lightly browned. Cut into wedges and serve at once.

SERVES: 4

CALORIES PER SERVING: 64

NUTRITION PER SERVING

Carbohydrate: ...... 2.5 g Cholesterol: .... .7 mg Potassium: .... 259 mg
Protein:.............. 5 g Fiber: .... .3 g Calcium:.......... 46 mg
Total Fat: .... 3.5 g Sodium: .... 78 mg Iron: .... 1 mg

Spinach Cheese Soufflé

1 package (10 ounce) frozen chopped spinach
1/2 cup 1% lowfat cottage cheese
1 scallion including top, thinly sliced
1/4 teaspoon nutmeg
1/8 teaspoon white pepper
2 egg whites

Cook spinach in a small amount of water and drain well. Add cottage cheese, scallion, nutmeg, and pepper. Beat egg whites until stiff peaks form; fold through spinach mixture. Pour into a nonstick baking dish. Bake in a 350° F oven 20 minutes, or until firm.

SERVES: 4

CALORIES PER SERVING: 44

NUTRITION PER SERVING

Carbohydrate: .... 3 g Cholesterol: .... 1 mg Potassium: .... 268 mg
Protein:.............. 7 g Fiber: .... .4 g Calcium:.......... 82 mg
Total Fat: .... .7 g Sodium: .... 58 mg Iron: .... 1.5 mg

Spinach Mushroom Salad

1 pound fresh spinach
1 clove garlic
1/2 small red onion, thinly sliced
6 large fresh mushrooms, thinly sliced
1/4 cup unsalted tomato juice

2 tablespoons olive oil
3 tablespoons red wine vinegar
½ teaspoon dry mustard
⅛ teaspoon pepper

Wash spinach several times, until rinsing water is clear. Trim stems. Rub salad bowl with cut clove of garlic; discard remaining garlic. Add spinach, onion and mushrooms. Separately, combine tomato juice, oil, vinegar, mustard, and pepper; pour over spinach. Toss well and serve.

SERVES: 8
CALORIES PER SERVING: 45

NUTRITION PER SERVING

Carbohydrate: .... 3 g	Cholesterol: .... none	Potassium: .... 209 mg
Protein: .... 2 g	Fiber: .... .4 g	Calcium: .... 44 mg
Total Fat: .... 3.5 g	Sodium: .... 52 mg	Iron: .... 1.2 mg

Tomatoes Vinaigrette

2 tablespoons light olive oil
2 tablespoons red wine vinegar
2 tablespoons fresh lemon juice
1 clove garlic, crushed
½ teaspoon dried basil
½ teaspoon dried thyme
1 teaspoon fresh chopped parsley
⅛ teaspoon ground white pepper
2 pints cherry tomatoes, stems removed

Combine olive oil, vinegar, lemon juice, garlic, basil, thyme, parsley, and pepper. Place tomatoes in a bowl and pour dressing over all. Toss lightly to coat well. Chill for several hours before serving.

SERVES: 8
CALORIES PER SERVING: 56

NUTRITION PER SERVING

Carbohydrate: .... 7 g	Cholesterol: .... none	Potassium: .... 313 mg
Protein: .... 2 g	Fiber: .... .7 g	Calcium: .... 17 mg
Total Fat: .... 3 g	Sodium: .... 4 mg	Iron: .... .6 mg

Herbed Cherry Tomatoes

1 cup cherry tomatoes

2 tablespoons lemon juice

1 teaspoon olive oil

¹/₄ teaspoon dried basil

¹/₄ teaspoon dried thyme

¹/₈ teaspoon garlic powder

1 tablespoon chopped fresh parsley

Wash tomatoes and remove stems; place in a bowl. Combine remaining ingredients; pour over tomatoes and toss lightly. Chill until ready to serve.

SERVES: 2

CALORIES PER SERVING: 48

NUTRITION PER SERVING

Carbohydrate: .... 7 g	Cholesterol: .... none	Potassium: .... 333 mg
Protein: .... 1 g	Fiber: .... .7 g	Calcium: .... 20 mg
Total Fat: .... 2 g	Sodium: .... 5 mg	Iron: .... .7 mg

9

Salad Dressings

Buttermilk Celery Seed Dressing

1 cup buttermilk
1 teaspoon lemon juice
1 teaspoon honey
½ teaspoon celery seed

Combine buttermilk, lemon juice, honey, and celery seed. Beat well. Refrigerate until ready to use.

YIELD: 1 Cup of Dressing
CALORIES PER TABLESPOON: 8

NUTRITION PER SERVING

Carbohydrate: ....1 g	Cholesterol: ....6 mg	Potassium: ....24 mg
Protein:.............5 g	Fiber: ....trace	Calcium:..........18 mg
Total Fat: ....1 g	Sodium: ....20 mg	Iron: ....trace

Cucumber Dill Salad Dressing

1¼ cups peeled, seeded, and sliced cucumber
¼ cup plain lowfat yogurt
2 tablespoons fresh lemon juice

1 teaspoon dried dillweed
¹/₂ teaspoon sugar
¹/₄ teaspoon onion powder
¹/₄ teaspoon garlic powder
¹/₈ teaspoon pepper

In the container of an electric blender or food processor, combine cucumber, yogurt, lemon juice, dill, sugar, onion and garlic powders, and pepper. Cover and blend until cucumber is pureed. Serve over mixed salad greens, sliced vegetables, or fish.

YIELD: 1 Cup of Dressing
CALORIES PER TABLESPOON: 5

NUTRITION PER SERVING

Carbohydrate: .... .96 g	Cholesterol: .... none	Potassium: .... 31 mg
Protein: .... .25 g	Fiber: .... none	Calcium: .... 10 mg
Total Fat: .... .06 g	Sodium: .... 3 mg	Iron: .... .06 mg

No-Oil Salad Dressing

2 ounces wine vinegar
4 ounces water
¹/₂ teaspoon frozen apple-juice concentrate
¹/₄ teaspoon oregano
¹/₈ teaspoon pepper

Combine all ingredients. Mix vigorously and pour over salad greens. Refrigerate leftovers.

YIELD: ¹/₃ Cup of Dressing
CALORIES PER TABLESPOON: 1

NUTRITION PER SERVING

Carbohydrate: .... .7 g	Cholesterol: .... none	Potassium: .... 7 mg
Protein: .... none	Fiber: .... none	Calcium: .... .7 mg
Total Fat: .... none	Sodium: .... none	Iron: .... .05 mg

Salt-Free Italian Dressing

¹/₂ cup salad oil
¹/₄ cup vinegar

¼ cup water
1 clove garlic, minced
¼ teaspoon cayenne pepper
¼ teaspoon dry mustard
¼ teaspoon oregano
1 teaspoon frozen apple-juice concentrate

Combine all ingredients in a cruet bottle. Shake well. Store in refrigerator until ready to serve.

YIELD: 1 Cup of Dressing
CALORIES PER TABLESPOON: 60

NUTRITION PER SERVING

Carbohydrate: .... .4 g	Cholesterol: .... none	Potassium: .... 5 mg
Protein:........... trace	Fiber: .... trace	Calcium:........... .4 mg
Total Fat: .... 6.8 g	Sodium: .... .06 mg	Iron: .... .03 mg

Tomato Juice Salad Dressing

1 cup salt-free tomato juice
¼ cup fresh lemon juice
2 tablespoons finely grated celery
1 clove garlic, finely minced
½ teaspoon dried oregano
¼ teaspoon pepper

Combine all ingredients in a jar. Shake vigorously and refrigerate several hours before using.

YIELD: 1⅓ Cups of Dressing
CALORIES PER TABLESPOON: 3

NUTRITION PER SERVING

Carbohydrate: .... .9 g	Cholesterol: .... none	Potassium: .... 36 mg
Protein:........... .09 g	Fiber: .... .07 g	Calcium:........... 2 mg
Total Fat: .... trace	Sodium: .... 1.3 mg	Iron: .... .06 mg

Tofu Roquefort Dressing

1 cup tofu
3 tablespoons vegetable oil

3 tablespoons vinegar
1 tablespoon honey
¹/₄ teaspoon garlic powder
¹/₈ teaspoon pepper
1 ounce Roquefort cheese, crumbled

Blend all but the cheese until smooth. Pour into a bowl and add crumbled Roquefort cheese. Serve with a fruit or vegetable salad bowl.

YIELD: 1½ Cups of Dressing
CALORIES PER TABLESPOON: 28

NUTRITION PER SERVING

Carbohydrate: .... 1 g	Cholesterol: .... .9 mg	Potassium: .... 5 mg
Protein: .... 1 g	Fiber: .... none	Calcium: .... 6 mg
Total Fat: .... 2.3 g	Sodium: .... .04 mg	Iron: .... .02 mg

── 10 ──

Breads and Desserts

Banana Raisin Bread

2 cups whole-wheat flour
1 cup yellow cornmeal
1 teaspoon baking soda
1 cup mashed ripe bananas
1 cup buttermilk
¾ cup unsulphured molasses
¾ cup seedless raisins

In a large bowl, mix together flour, cornmeal, and baking soda. Stir in mashed bananas, buttermilk, molasses, and raisins. Turn into 2 nonstick, 9 × 4–inch loaf pans. Bake in a preheated 350° F oven 45 minutes. Cool 10 minutes, turn out of pans onto a wire rack. Loaves may be wrapped in foil and frozen.

YIELD: 2 Loaves of 10 Slices Each
CALORIES PER SERVING: 123

NUTRITION PER SERVING

Carbohydrate: ....28 g	Cholesterol: .... .4 mg	Potassium: ....275 mg
Protein:..............3 g	Fiber: .... 1.4 g	Calcium:.......... 45 mg
Total Fat: ....5 g	Sodium: .... 20 mg	Iron: .... 1.3 mg

Oatmeal Raisin Muffins

1½ cups unbleached flour
½ cup brown sugar
2½ teaspoons baking powder
¾ teaspoon baking soda
¼ cup corn oil
¾ cup raw oatmeal
¼ cup raisins
1¼ cups buttermilk
1 egg white, slightly beaten

Combine flour, sugar, baking powder, and baking soda. Add corn oil and stir with a fork until the mixture looks like coarse meal. Stir in oats. Add raisins. Add buttermilk and egg white; stir just to moisten dry ingredients. Fill paper-lined muffin pan cups about two-thirds full. Bake at 425° F for 20 to 25 minutes, or until lightly browned.

SERVES: 12
CALORIES PER SERVING: 151

NUTRITION PER SERVING

Carbohydrate: .... 24 g	Cholesterol: .... .9 mg	Potassium: .... 121 mg
Protein: .... 3 g	Fiber: .... .07 g	Calcium: .... 42 mg
Total Fat: .... 4.8 g	Sodium: .... 142 mg	Iron: .... .9 mg

Date and Nut Muffins

1 package (8 ounce) pitted dates, chopped
¼ teaspoon baking soda
½ cup boiling water
1 egg white
¼ cup corn oil
1½ cups unbleached flour
⅓ cup light brown sugar
¼ cup chopped nuts
½ teaspoon vanilla extract

Combine dates and baking soda in a large bowl. Add boiling water, stir, and set aside. Beat together the egg white and corn oil; gradually stir into the date mixture. Separately, combine flour, sugar, and nuts; add to batter. Add vanilla and stir just until dry ingredients are moistened. Pour into paper-lined muffin pans, filling cups two-thirds full. Bake in a 375° F oven for 25 minutes, or until golden brown.

SERVES: 12

CALORIES PER SERVING: 183

NUTRITION PER SERVING

Carbohydrate: ....29 g Cholesterol: .... 23 mg Potassium: .... 149 mg
Protein:..............9 g Fiber: ....4 g Calcium:.......... 19 mg
Total Fat: .... 6.9 g Sodium: .... 7 mg Iron: .... 1.3 mg

Graham Carrot Muffins

1 cup graham or whole-wheat flour
1 cup unbleached flour
³/₄ cup coarsely grated carrots
¹/₄ cup brown sugar
1 tablespoon baking powder
1 teaspoon salt
1 teaspoon grated orange rind
1 cup skim milk
¹/₄ cup corn oil
¹/₄ cup molasses
2 egg whites

Combine graham flour, unbleached flour, carrots, brown sugar, baking powder, salt, and orange rind; mix well. In a small bowl, combine the milk, oil, molasses, and egg whites; beat well. Add the liquid ingredients to the dry ingredients, stirring just until combined. Fill nonstick muffin cups or paper liners about three-quarters full. Bake in a 400° F oven for 20 minutes, or until lightly browned.

SERVES: 12

CALORIES PER SERVING: 157

NUTRITION PER SERVING

Carbohydrate: ....25 g Cholesterol: .... .3 mg Potassium: .... 188 mg
Protein:............ 3.6 g Fiber: .... 1.1 g Calcium:.......... 49 mg
Total Fat: .... 4.8 g Sodium: .... 25 mg Iron: .... 1.1 mg

Whole-Wheat Soda Bread

1 pound whole-wheat flour
¹/₈ teaspoon salt

1 teaspoon baking soda
1 teaspoon baking powder
1½ cups skim milk

Set aside one cup of flour. Sift remaining flour, salt, baking soda, and baking powder into a mixing bowl. Make a well in the center and pour in the milk. Gradually mix in reserved cup of flour. The dough should be moist, so use more liquid if necessary. Turn onto a floured board and knead lightly to form a loaf to fit a nonstick 8½ × 4½–inch loaf pan, or form a round cake to bake on a flat nonstick baking sheet. Cut a deep cross in the center of the loaf. Bake in a 400° F oven for 30 to 40 minutes.

YIELD: 16 Half-Inch Slices
CALORIES PER SERVING: 118

NUTRITION PER SERVING

Carbohydrate: ....12 g	Cholesterol: .... .4 mg	Potassium: .... 94 mg
Protein:........... 2.7 g	Fiber: .... 1.5 g	Calcium:.......... 38 mg
Total Fat: ....7 g	Sodium: .... 33 mg	Iron: .... .5 mg

Raisin Honey Rye Bread

1 cup rye flour
1 cup unbleached flour
1½ teaspoons baking powder
1 teaspoon baking soda
1 teaspoon salt
½ teaspoon ginger
½ teaspoon cinnamon
1 cup skim milk
½ cup honey
¼ cup corn oil
2 egg whites
½ cup seedless raisins

Combine the two flours, baking powder, baking soda, salt, ginger, and cinnamon; stir together. In a small bowl, combine the milk, honey, corn oil, and egg whites; beat well. Add liquid ingredients to dry ingredients and stir until just combined. Add raisins and stir through. Pour batter into a nonstick 8½ × 4½–inch loaf pan. Bake in a 350° F oven for 45 to 50 minutes, or until top is lightly browned.

YIELD: 16 Half-Inch Slices
CALORIES PER SERVING: 138

NUTRITION PER SERVING

Carbohydrate:	24 g	Cholesterol:	.2 mg	Potassium:	107 mg
Protein:	3 g	Fiber:	.8 g	Calcium:	32 mg
Total Fat:	3.6 g	Sodium:	47 mg	Iron:	.7 mg

Baked Apple with Lemon Raisin Topping

4 medium baking apples
4 teaspoons frozen apple-juice concentrate
¼ teaspoon cinnamon
⅛ teaspoon nutmeg
4 tablespoons lowfat lemon yogurt
2 teaspoons seedless white raisins

Core apples from stem side almost through the other side. Remove pits. Remove ½-inch of apple peel from the top. Fill each apple cavity with 1 teaspoon frozen apple-juice concentrate. Sprinkle with cinnamon and nutmeg. Place in a small baking dish. Pour ½-inch water around apples. Bake at 350° F for 20 minutes, or until apples are soft but still holding their shape. Serve warm or cold with a topping of lemon yogurt and a sprinkling of raisins.

SERVES: 4
CALORIES PER SERVING: 144

NUTRITION PER SERVING

Carbohydrate:	35 g	Cholesterol:	1 mg	Potassium:	290 mg
Protein:	.7 g	Fiber:	2.2 g	Calcium:	43 mg
Total Fat:	1.2 g	Sodium:	10 mg	Iron:	.7 mg

Poached Apples

3 large yellow or green apples
1 cup apple juice
1 teaspoon lemon juice
1 teaspoon honey
¼ teaspoon cinnamon

Cut each apple in half, through the "equator" line. Peel and scoop out seeds, using a melon scoop. Place in a large skillet, round side up. Add apple juice, lemon juice, honey, and cinnamon. Cover and simmer over low heat until apples are just tender but still holding their shape. Chill in juice until ready to serve.

SERVES: 6

CALORIES PER SERVING: 86

NUTRITION PER SERVING

Carbohydrate: .... 21 g	Cholesterol: .... none	Potassium: .... 160 mg
Protein: .... trace	Fiber: .... 1 g	Calcium: .... 10 mg
Total Fat: .... .5 g	Sodium: .... 1 mg	Iron: .... .5 mg

Poached Pears

6 small, almost ripe pears
1 cup orange juice
1 teaspoon vanilla extract
1 tablespoon frozen apple-juice concentrate

Pare the pears, slice in half lengthwise, and scoop out seeds with a melon scoop. Place pear halves in a single layer in a large skillet. Add orange juice, vanilla, and apple-juice concentrate. Cover and simmer over low heat until pears are just tender but still holding their shape. Chill in juice until ready to serve.

SERVES: 6

CALORIES PER SERVING: 122

NUTRITION PER SERVING

Carbohydrate: .... 30 g	Cholesterol: .... none	Potassium: .... 303 mg
Protein: .... 1 g	Fiber: .... 2 g	Calcium: .... 18 mg
Total Fat: .... 1 g	Sodium: .... .03 mg	Iron: .... .6 mg

Banana Orange Amandine

2 oranges, peeled, sliced in thick circles
2 bananas, cut in 1-inch chunks
1/2 cup seedless white raisins
1 cup plain nonfat yogurt
1 teaspoon vanilla extract
2 tablespoons soft brown sugar
2 tablespoons slivered almonds

274

Arrange orange slices in a nonstick flat baking dish. Add banana chunks between oranges. Scatter raisins over all. Combine yogurt and vanilla; spoon in a thin layer over the arranged fruit. Sprinkle with brown sugar and almonds. Broil 4 inches from heat until sugar carmelizes. Serve at once.

SERVES: 6

CALORIES PER SERVING: 133

NUTRITION PER SERVING

Carbohydrate: ....30 g	Cholesterol: .... .3 mg	Potassium: .... 411 mg
Protein:.............3 g	Fiber: ....6 g	Calcium:.......... 76 mg
Total Fat: .... 1.5 g	Sodium: .... 5 mg	Iron: .... 1.1 mg

Fresh Fruit Delight

1 banana, sliced
½ cantaloupe, cut into 1-inch chunks
1 kiwifruit, peeled and sliced thin
1 cup plain nonfat yogurt
¼ teaspoon ground nutmeg
1 teaspoon grated orange rind
½ teaspoon vanilla extract

Combine all fruit and spoon into 6 stemmed sherbet glasses. Separately, combine yogurt, nutmeg, orange rind, and vanilla; spoon over fruit. Top with a dash of nutmeg.

SERVES: 6

CALORIES PER SERVING: 51

NUTRITION PER SERVING

Carbohydrate: ....10 g	Cholesterol: .... .7 mg	Potassium: .... 281 mg
Protein:............ 2.6 g	Fiber: ....1 g	Calcium:.......... 83 mg
Total Fat: .... trace	Sodium: .... 5 mg	Iron: .... .03 mg

Broiled Honeyed Bananas

2 bananas
1 tablespoon lemon juice
2 teaspoons honey

Peel bananas and cut in half lengthwise; if very long, cut in half crosswise as well. Sprinkle with lemon juice and arrange in a buttered baking pan with rounded sides up; brush with honey. Broil for 5 minutes, or until lightly browned.

SERVES: 2

CALORIES PER SERVING: 124

NUTRITION PER SERVING

Carbohydrate:	32 g	Cholesterol:	none	Potassium:	454 mg
Protein:	1 g	Fiber:	.6 g	Calcium:	11 mg
Total Fat:	trace	Sodium:	1 mg	Iron:	.8 mg

Prune Apricot Compote

1 pound dried prunes and apricots
1 tablespoon honey
1 tablespoon grated lemon rind
1/2 teaspoon cinnamon
1/4 teaspoon nutmeg
2 tablespoons cornstarch
1/2 cup orange juice

Cover dried fruits with cold water and let stand at room temperature for several hours. Drain off water and measure 1 cup of it; pour into saucepan. Add honey, lemon rind, cinnamon, and nutmeg. Bring to a boil and cook for 10 minutes. Separately, stir cornstarch into orange juice until smooth; slowly add to cooked syrup. Add dried reserved fruits. Cook over low heat and stir until sauce is thickened. Serve hot or cold.

SERVES: 8

CALORIES PER SERVING: 81

NUTRITION PER SERVING

Carbohydrate:	21 g	Cholesterol:	none	Potassium:	219 mg
Protein:	.9 g	Fiber:	.6 g	Calcium:	15 mg
Total Fat:	.2 g	Sodium:	4 mg	Iron:	1.1 mg

Orange Sherbet

1/2 cup nonfat dry milk solids
1 tablespoon fresh lemon juice
1 teaspoon almond flavoring
1/2 cup water
1 can (6 ounce) frozen orange-juice concentrate

¾ cup water
¼ cup frozen apple-juice concentrate
2 egg whites

Place milk solids, lemon juice, almond flavoring, and ½ cup water in a mixing bowl; beat until mixture is thick and fluffy. Add frozen orange-juice concentrate; beat again. Add ¾ cup water and frozen apple-juice concentrate; beat again. Pour mixture into two ice-cube trays with separators removed. When mixture is partially frozen, remove and beat again. Beat egg whites until stiff peaks form; fold through orange mixture. Return to freezing compartment until frozen firmly.

SERVES: 8

CALORIES PER SERVING: 76

NUTRITION PER SERVING

Carbohydrate: .... 16 g Cholesterol: .... .7 mg Potassium: .... 297 mg
Protein: .... 3 g Fiber: .... .07 g Calcium: .... 64 mg
Total Fat: .... trace Sodium: .... 70 mg Iron: .... .2 mg

Ricotta Tofu Pudding

½ cup lowfat ricotta cheese
1 cup drained tofu
½ cup plain nonfat yogurt
½ cup carob chips
3 tablespoons chopped walnuts

Place cheese and tofu into a deep bowl. Beat until light and fluffy. Add yogurt and beat well. Melt carob chips in the top of a double boiler over hot water; add to cheese mixture. Spoon into pudding dishes and top with chopped nuts.

SERVES: 4

CALORIES PER SERVING: 128

NUTRITION PER SERVING

Carbohydrate: .... 16 g Cholesterol: ...... 9.5 mg Potassium: .... 65 mg
Protein: .... 7 g Fiber: .... 1.4 g Calcium: .... 84 mg
Total Fat: .... 7.2 g Sodium: .... .2 mg Iron: .... .5 mg

Nutty Carob Drops

5 cups grape-nut flakes cereal
2 cups carob chips
3 tablespoons chunky peanut butter
¼ cup seedless raisins

Place grape-nut flakes cereal in a large bowl. Put carob chips and peanut butter into the top of a double boiler. Melt over boiling water, stirring constantly until well combined. Spoon mixture into grape-nut flakes and mix well. Add raisins. Drop by teaspoonfuls on a sheet of wax paper. Allow to firm up.

YIELD: 36 cookies
CALORIES PER SERVING: 38

NUTRITION PER SERVING

Carbohydrate: .... 10 g	Cholesterol: .... none	Potassium: .... 27 mg
Protein: .... 1 g	Fiber: .... .7 g	Calcium: .... 3 mg
Total Fat: .... .7 g	Sodium: .... 51 mg	Iron: .... .7 mg

Carrot Cookies

½ cup oil
½ cup honey
2 egg whites
1 cup whole-wheat flour
½ cup wheat germ
½ cup nonfat dry milk
1 teaspoon baking powder
½ teaspoon cinnamon
1 cup grated carrots
½ cup raisins
¼ cup chopped nuts
1 teaspoon vanilla

Beat oil, honey, and egg whites together. Separately, combine flour, wheat germ, dry milk, baking powder, and cinnamon; add to batter. Add carrots, raisins, nuts, and vanilla. Mix well. Drop by teaspoonfuls on two nonstick cookie sheets. Bake in a 350° F oven for 12 to 15 minutes.

YIELD: 36 Cookies
CALORIES PER SERVING: 75

Carbohydrate: .... 9 g	Cholesterol: .... .2 mg	Potassium: .... 76 mg
Protein:............ 1.6 g	Fiber: .... .4 g	Calcium:.......... 18 mg
Total Fat: .... 3.8 g	Sodium: .... 19 mg	Iron: .... .4 mg

Carrot Raisin Date Cookies

½ cup cooked and mashed carrots
1 teaspoon grated orange rind
1 teaspoon lemon juice
2 stiffly beaten egg whites
1 cup unbleached flour
1 teaspoon baking powder
½ teaspoon ginger
¼ teaspoon nutmeg
⅓ cup raisins
⅓ cup chopped dates

Combine mashed carrots, orange rind, and lemon juice. Fold through stiffly beaten egg whites. Separately, combine flour, baking powder, ginger, and nutmeg; fold through batter. Carefully add raisins and dates. Drop by teaspoonfuls onto a nonstick cookie sheet. Bake in a 350° F oven for 12 minutes, or until lightly browned around the edges.

YIELD: 2 Dozen Cookies

CALORIES PER SERVING: 34

Carbohydrate: .... 7 g	Cholesterol: .... none	Potassium: .... 48 mg
Protein:............. 9 g	Fiber: .... .1 g	Calcium:.......... 7 mg
Total Fat: .... .04 g	Sodium: .... 19 mg	Iron: .... .3 mg

Apple Carob Brownies

½ cup oil
½ cup honey
4 egg whites
1 teaspoon vanilla
1 cup unbleached flour
1 cup whole-wheat flour

2 teaspoons baking powder
½ teaspoon salt
½ cup carob powder
½ cup chopped nuts
½ cup seedless raisins
1 cup grated fresh-peeled apple

Beat oil, honey, and egg whites together. Add vanilla and beat until smooth. Sift both types of flour, baking powder, and salt into a bowl; gradually stir into batter. Add carob powder, nuts, raisins, and grated apple. Mix well. Pour into a nonstick 9 × 13–inch pan. Bake in a 350° F oven for 30 minutes, or until lightly browned. Cool in the pan and then cut into squares.

SERVES: 24
CALORIES PER SERVING: 129

NUTRITION PER SERVING

Carbohydrate: ....17 g	Cholesterol: .... none	Potassium: ....76 mg
Protein:..............2 g	Fiber: ....6 g	Calcium:..........11 mg
Total Fat: ....6.2 g	Sodium: ....37 mg	Iron: ....6 mg

Honey Oatmeal Bars

2 cups uncooked oatmeal
¾ cup unbleached flour
¾ cup whole-wheat flour
½ cup corn oil
½ cup honey
½ cup chopped nuts
1 teaspoon cinnamon
¼ teaspoon nutmeg
¼ teaspoon salt

Combine all ingredients in a large bowl. Beat at low speed of electric mixer until mixture is crumbly. Spread over bottom of a nonstick 9 × 13–inch pan. Bake in a 375° F oven for 25 minutes. Cool and cut into 2-inch squares.

SERVES: 24
CALORIES PER SERVING: 156

NUTRITION PER SERVING

Carbohydrate: ....14 g	Cholesterol: .... trace	Potassium: ....45 mg
Protein:............ 1.9 g	Fiber: ....5 g	Calcium:..........4 mg
Total Fat: .... 10.9 g	Sodium: ....44 mg	Iron: ....5 mg

INDEX